DETOX YOUR LIFE

A PRACTICAL GUIDE TO DETOXING YOUR BODY, MIND, HOME, AND RELATIONSHIPS

REBECCA CLIO GOULD

ELEMENTAL HARMONY PRESS

Grateful acknowledgment is made to the following for permission to reprint previously published material:

Marcia Baczynski: for permission to quote from "12 Ways To Say No Gracefully (Without Saying "Maybe Later")"

Notice: Mention of specific companies, organizations, or authorities in this book does not imply endorsement by the publisher, nor does mention of specific companies, organizations, or authorities imply that they endorse this book. Web addresses provided in this book were accurate at the time of publication.

The information contained in this book is intended to be educational and not for diagnosis, prescriptions, or treatment of any physical or mental health disorder whatsoever. This information should not replace consultation with a competent healthcare professional. The content in this book is intended to be used as an adjunct to a rational and responsible healthcare program prescribed by a professional healthcare practitioner. The author and publisher are in no way liable for any misuse of the material.

Edited by the Blue Garret
Design and composition by the Blue Garret
Cover design by Constance Mears
Author photo by Sharon Smith

Published by Elemental Harmony Press
P.O. Box 33433
Seattle, WA 98133

ISBN: 978-0-9976645-1-5 (paper)
ISBN: 978-0-9976645-2-2 (ebook)

Dedicated to you.

CONTENTS

START HERE

A FEW YEARS ago while writing my first book, *The Multi-Orgasmic Diet,* the words "detox your life" came to mind while I was brainstorming chapter titles. Why? Because *The Multi-Orgasmic Diet* is not really a diet book; it's a lifestyle book about how to feel more fulfilled by living your life with orgasmic energy flowing through you, all throughout your day. So, naturally, I was thinking about what gets in the way of feeling as energized, vibrant, and fulfilled as we yearn to be.

And one thing that came to mind was toxicity—in our bodies, in our minds, in our relationships. Toxicity gunks up our energy flow, weighs us down, and holds us back from feeling our best. But since this is such a vast subject, I decided the concept of *detoxing your life* deserved its own book, not just a chapter. So here we are.

Or at least that's why I'm here, writing this.

But why are you here, reading this?

Have you been feeling sluggish, drained, weighed down, overwhelmed, or just *blah*? Are you in a "toxic relationship" or find that you keep attracting "toxic" people into your life? Do you feel like there's some icky or sticky energy or something

bringing you down and keeping you stuck? Are you tired of
negative thought patterns getting in your way? Are you interested in how to have a cleaner diet or how to reduce toxic products in your environment? Do you want to feel more energetic
and optimistic, healthier and happier in body, mind, and spirit?

If you answered yes to even just one of those questions,
then you're in the right place. If you want to have more energy,
experience more flow in your life, and have healthier, happier
interactions with others and with your own self, then *Detox
Your Life* is a good starter guide.

In the following pages you'll learn about cleaning and
clearing your body, your mind, your energy, your home, and
your relationships so that you can feel your best—and, therefore, live your best life. Each chapter will contain practical
suggestions and activities to help you detox your body and
mind, declutter your home, and improve your relationships.
And at the end we'll take a look at the big picture; I'll show you
how to put it all together, how to weave it into your life in a
manageable way.

But What Does It Mean to "Detox" Your Life?

It means cleaning up and clearing out anything harmful to
your body, mind, and overall well-being. It means making
space for more of what you want. It means helping your body
and mind function as optimally as they can. This book is about
how to rid yourself of toxicity and clutter—both material and
non-material—so that you can have more energy, more joy, and
happier, healthier relationships.

Please note, though, that this is not meant to be a *comprehensive* detox guide. As a holistic health and resilience coach,
energy worker, and qigong teacher, I am simply sharing some
of the things I've seen work well, both in my personal and
professional experience over the years. I will be keeping this

simple, and using a "less is more" approach, because that's part of what detoxing your life is all about: freeing up your energy by removing excess and keeping the information clean and clear in order to reduce overwhelm and confusion.

And if you have some serious health conditions that could benefit from more comprehensive and in-depth physical and environmental detox processes? Please see the Resources section while also knowing that this book can still help you feel better, because detoxing is about more than just what we put into and onto our bodies. It's about the thoughts we think. It's about our beliefs. Our words. Our actions. Our environment. Our relationships.

Because this book covers these various subjects, you may think that not everything here applies to you. Maybe you are only interested in detoxing your physical body. Or maybe that's the one chapter you don't care about. In that case, you have the option of just turning to the chapters that *do* call to you. But I strongly encourage you to read the whole book. It's a quick read. And you just might discover something that resonates and helps you where you least expected. Plus, everything is connected. For example, the Mind chapter will assist you with the relationship stuff—and really with everything.

But before we go any further, let's clarify some terms.

Defining 'Toxic' and 'Detox'

As much as I love the sound of "Detox Your Life"—and it made sense to me the moment those words first went through my head—I must admit I spent some time reconsidering the title. I wondered if using the word "toxic" could be problematic, because it has such a negative connotation and tends to be overused, especially when talking about relationships. But rather than run from that word to avoid a possible misunderstanding, I'd rather clearly define and reframe it. And if even after reading my take on it you prefer to use some other word? Go for it.

Toxic is defined in the Oxford dictionary as "poisonous." But that's too extreme for the purposes of this book. So let's look at the synonyms, which include "harmful, dangerous, destructive, unsafe, environmentally unfriendly." My take on it is that toxicity, in general, is about harm. Maybe it won't kill you, but it's not good for you. And it's taking a toll or wreaking some sort of havoc, even if you're not totally aware of it.

Although most detoxes are about what we eat and drink, what we eat and drink are not the only sources of harm. Our thoughts can be harmful. What we talk about, what we read, what we watch on TV can be harmful. Relationships can be harmful. Although there are some foods and products that are toxic in the poisonous sense, most of this book will be referring to toxicity that is not deadly but that is harmful, destructive, or unfriendly.

Not all of this book is about dealing with what most people would consider "toxic." It's not all about addressing *obvious* harm. Sometimes it's subtle. And oftentimes small changes make a big difference. For example, we'll look at cleaning up and clearing out your physical environment for better energy flow. Household clutter isn't toxic in a poisonous way, but it can be "unfriendly"; it can take a toll and be harmful or destructive in subtle ways. So, we'll be looking at whatever in your life is blocking you, draining you, or depleting you physically, emotionally, mentally, or energetically so that you can feel healthier inside and out—feel lighter and brighter in every way, in every part of your life.

As for defining "detox," the Oxford dictionary definition is "a process or period of time in which one abstains from or rids the body of toxic or unhealthy substances." I extend this to go beyond just the body. I extend this definition to include unhealthy, self-limiting, havoc-wreaking thoughts and beliefs, as well as any physical clutter or problematic relationship dynamics. As mentioned above, detoxing can include decluttering to enhance energy flow and overall well-being. It also includes changing your thoughts and beliefs so that they are no longer toxic or contributing to toxicity. For example, sometimes all that needs to change is how we think of something or someone, rather than removing them from our lives.

"Toxic" may feel like an overstatement for some of what we will be addressing here, so take it or leave it. I also don't want you to feel even worse by viewing certain things or people in your life as "toxic," so let's keep that in check throughout the book—and throughout our lives. We don't want to demonize ourselves or others, or overuse the word "toxic," because *that* is actually quite harmful itself.

What matters to me is that using the word "toxic" doesn't feel bad to you. Perhaps it's best to focus less on labeling things or people as toxic, and instead focus more on the *de*toxing—on the cleaning up and clearing out anything physical or mental that is harming you and preventing you from feeling your very best and living the life you want.

You can even think of it more like *cleaning* your body, your mind, your energy, your relationships, and your home environments in order to clear out any negativity, any heaviness, anything blocking your energy flow or draining you.

To summarize, my definitions are as follows:

Toxic: Anything material or non-material that is harmful to your physical and emotional well-being, to your holistic health. Anything that drains your energy, holds you back, gets in the way of you feeling your best and living a fulfilling and healthy life.

Detox: Totally abstaining from, or limiting exposure to, whatever is toxic in your life, whatever is draining you, clogging the pipes, blocking the flow.

In order to feel your absolute best—physically, mentally,

emotionally, and energetically—you need to be honest about what is in your way, what is stopping you, what is weighing you down or depleting you. When you're able to honestly identify your blockages, that's when you can remove them. Through the process of detoxing your life, you can reduce or eliminate suffering by letting go of what's not serving you—and by bringing in more of what's good for you.

How Toxic Are You?

Yikes! What an awful question. But it's a question I was considering asking. I was considering giving you a quiz or self-assessment to take because that's the kind of thing books like this often include in order to highlight your pain points to convince you that you need the solutions offered in the book.

But guess what? I don't want you thinking of yourself as toxic. I don't want to "program" you to view yourself as toxic. I don't want to scare you into thinking you need this. I just want to offer you this opportunity to identify what's going on in your life that needs some detoxing. And I want to provide some suggestions on how to clean up whatever needs to be cleaned up in both your inner and outer worlds.

Some people are only motivated by fear to make changes. But I don't want to manipulate you by using fear tactics. I'd rather just present some information and ideas for you to consider—and hopefully also inspire and encourage you to make changes coming from a place of love. A place of self-love. Loving yourself so much that you want to feel your best and are willing to do whatever it takes, whether it's baby steps or big dramatic shifts all at once.

So let's skip this step of a quiz or self-assessment designed to convince you just how much or how little you need to do here. You don't need that. All you need is to commit to a few hours to read this all the way through with an open mind and a willingness to look honestly at what's happening, and not happening, in your life. And the willingness to follow some, if not all, of the suggestions in this book so that you can feel lighter and brighter, healthier and happier.

Sound good?

Now, let's continue with a better question...

How Are You Feeling?

This is always a good question to ask. Our feelings are messengers. It's wise to pay attention to them and to recognize that we have the power to change how we feel if we don't like how we feel. And my guess is that you started reading this book because you want to feel better. But feel better in what way? Feel better how?

Have you been feeling sluggish or heavy? Low energy? Depleted? Drained? Concerned about health problems? Taken advantage of? Stagnant or stuck? Overwhelmed? Anxious? Irritable? Down on yourself? Overly confrontational or overly avoidant in dealing with "difficult people"?

You're not alone.

The truth is, at the time of writing the first draft of this book, I was coming out of a long stretch of not feeling so great and recognizing some toxicity—some harm—coming from my own thoughts and from various types of relationships. I tend to eat pretty healthy and have a fairly non-toxic living environment. But some of my thought patterns and some of the people in my life? Well, let's just say there was quite a bit of heaviness, energy drain, stagnation, pain, and limitations on and off over the couple of years prior to when I started writing this book. And I'm happy to report that by going through my own process of detoxing my life, I made some huge shifts in cleaning up and clearing out life-sucking thought patterns. I also distanced myself from certain people and learned how to disengage from toxic relationships.

So I am here to say that change for the better is absolutely 100 percent possible. And I am here as your guide for whatever changes would serve you best. As for how to figure out what needs changing? You can start with looking at how you are feeling now versus how you *want* to feel.

Go ahead and write it down.

What are your goals? What do you want? How do you want to feel? Put it in writing now, or come back to this later. But be sure to write it down. Being able to visually see this stuff in writing will help you act on it. It will also ensure that you don't forget what your goals are!

Breaking Bad Habits

One thing we'll be doing here is breaking bad habits by creating new, healthier habits. Humans tend to get addicted, or get in the habit of thinking about, talking about, or wanting what we know is not so good for us—or at least what's not best for us.

We may be in the habit of commiserating and complaining as a way of bonding. We may get hooked on unhealthy foods, drugs, and alcohol to self-medicate or fill a void—or simply because it tastes or feels good. We may get addicted to *people* and find ourselves attracted to and getting stuck in relationships with people who don't treat us well—or who just aren't the best fit. We may be in the habit of thinking self-limiting, self-defeating thoughts. *Why do we do this?*

We are creatures of habit, as well as creatures who long to belong. We are susceptible to direct marketing tactics and peer pressure, as well as indirect, unspoken influences—just going along with what others are doing. It takes conscious effort and conscious choice to break habits, to choose healthier options,

START HERE   9

to make changes. It requires committing to what we most want for ourselves, giving what we *want* more attention than what we *don't* want.

The habit of thinking negatively or giving more attention to what does *not* feel good is a habit that must be broken for optimal well-being. But people often say that habits are hard to break. That's what many believe. So, what if we start off by changing *that* belief and saying it doesn't have to be so hard? It just requires conscious awareness, clear intention, subconscious reprogramming (more on that later!), and a commitment to make changes that will set you up for success.

Keep in mind that there are ways of breaking habits that can be relatively easy and fun, like listening to some hypnotic meditation as you go to sleep or setting up a reward system or trading out the bad habit for something good, something healthy, enjoyable, pleasurable. For example, what if every time you caught yourself about to check email or social media again, in an excessive or habitual way, you instead danced around to your favorite song or gave yourself a hug?

Get creative and playful with breaking habits. Crowd out bad habits with good ones. But first of all, identify what is underlying the habit and the benefits of breaking it. This can keep you motivated and clear about sticking with your commitment.

It can take time to replace unhealthy habits, so be patient and gentle with yourself. If it's something you've been doing for years, then it might take more than the typical twenty-one or twenty-eight days we often hear about—or the more recently discovered average of sixty-six days to break an old habit or create a new one. It also might *not* take as long! Be open to the possibility that change can happen quickly, but don't get discouraged if it takes longer.

To set yourself up for success with detoxing your life, it is essential that you commit to breaking bad habits and creating healthier ones. You can use these steps to get started:

Steps for breaking a habit or addiction:

1. Identify the habit or addiction.
2. Identify how it's toxic or harmful.
3. List the benefits of quitting it.
4. Identify changes to make in your environment that will set you up for success (for example, get rid of sugary products or put them on a shelf that's too high to reach if you're cutting out sugar).
5. Come up with a few things you can do each day to crowd out the habit and/or reward yourself.
6. Commit to a certain number of days, weeks, or months to prioritize making this change.
7. Tell at least one other person. Accountability and support is helpful. If you're feeling hesitant to tell someone you know, feel free to send me a confidential message via my website: www.rebeccacliogould.com/contact.

Note: You can use a similar process for creating new habits —obviously you'd list the benefits of starting instead of quitting, and there'd be no list of harm, unless you want to identify the harm in *not* developing the healthy habit.

There's a bonus worksheet at www.rebeccacliogould.com/detoxbonuses to support you with this process, as well as goal-setting. And I suggest you take that step, with or without the worksheet, before diving into the next chapter. But first, a little note about energy.

What's Energy Have to Do with This?

It's all energy. Everything is energy. And as both a qigong teacher and a health coach, a common question I hear, and have asked plenty of times myself, is, "How can I have *more* energy?"

One of the main goals of any type of detox is to have more —and better—energy.

People also often tell me that I "have great energy," and so this book is an opportunity for me to share with you how I take care of myself in order to have such "great energy."

What's my secret? Well, my main one is no secret. It's qigong (vital life force energy cultivation, pronounced "chee kung") and meditation, especially Sheng Zhen (pronounced "shung jen"), which includes heart-opening energy cultivation and meditation practices. Qigong is an awesome practice for detoxing your life, because it basically is an energy detox. Just like you need to drink water every day and urinate every day, qigong is a daily process for bringing in fresh, pure qi (energy) and sending out stagnant, murky qi. And Sheng Zhen has the added bonus of being extra good for your heart and your emotions, so I'll share more on that with you later.

In addition to my Sheng Zhen practice, my relatively clean diet and home contribute to the quality and level of my energy. I also have a high level of self-awareness and consistently correct harmful ways of thinking. My boundaries in personal and professional contexts also serve me by preventing and/or repairing energy drains. All of these are important factors. And that's why this detox book is taking a holistic approach. We cannot expect a traditional detox to result in optimal well-being by only addressing what we do or don't ingest.

Energy depletion is a common problem, whether it's because of poor diet, toxic relationships, negative thinking, or some combination of those and other drains. And this book can help. After experiencing things beyond my control that zapped or tainted my energy—such as a nearly fatal car accident as a teenager and some relational trauma as a young adult —I've done my best to focus more on what I *can* control when it comes to the quantity and quality of my energy. Based on personal and professional experience, I'll share ways for you to increase your energy as well as how to protect, replenish, and enhance the quality of your energy. First we'll begin by looking at what you put into your BODY, but it won't stop there. It's just the beginning.

Next we will explore the MIND—our thinking, our words. After that, we'll focus on your HOME environment, mostly looking at decluttering as a form of detox but also touching upon getting rid of toxic cleaning and body-care products. And then, RELATIONSHIPS. Although you *can* pick and choose which chapters to read, I suggest reading them all, because there's definitely some overlap. And at the end, I'll show you how to put it all together with a ten-day sample plan.

My Philosophy

I truly believe that we all deserve to have the energy and health and fulfilling life that we want. I believe we are affected not only by what we put into our bodies, but also by what we put *on* our bodies, who we interact with and how, our home environment, our work environment, other people's energy and words, and the thoughts and beliefs in our own heads. And I believe that we have the power to consciously detox our lives. This happens not only by eliminating certain things and people from our lives, but also by cleaning up our thoughts, energy, and our ways of relating and communicating with ourselves and others. This book will help get you started with all of that.

So, are you ready to detox your life?

Let's do this.

BODY

WHY BEGIN WITH THE BODY? Our physical bodies are with us 24/7. Our bodies are our temples. And usually when we hear the word "detox," we think it's going to be about what we eat and drink, what we physically consume. So why not start here?

Although making dietary changes can be challenging, it can also be a great place to start. It's straightforward, feels empowering, and you can begin to notice benefits pretty quickly. That being said, if you'd rather begin with detoxing other aspects of your life, or don't feel that you need to implement the suggestions in this chapter, that's fine.

But let's check in with the body first.

How are you feeling in your body these days? Do you feel weighed down or sluggish? Weak or inflexible? How's your digestion? Your bowel movements? Your energy level? What's happening with your skin?

What we put into our bodies, as well as what we put *on* our bodies, what we ingest, inhale, and absorb, can greatly impact how we feel—not just physically, but also emotionally and energetically. This chapter primarily focuses on what we put *in* our bodies. In the Home chapter, we will look at what we put *on* our bodies (for example, body-care products) as well as what we inhale, such as through cleaning products and polluted air. As always, some of this book's content may apply to your life and some may not. Pick and choose what needs detoxing.

If you know your diet could use some cleaning up, or if you simply aren't feeling your very best, starting with a physical detox could make a noticeable difference. Oftentimes even just the smallest adjustments, like drinking more water, can have a big impact. And sometimes it takes more extreme measures.

Your path will depend on where you are currently, as well as where you want to be. You'll need to decide what you want, how you want to feel, and what it's going to take to get you there. And since we are all unique individuals, there's not one right path for every person. Part of this *Detox Your Life* experience will be about experimenting. Seeing what works. Seeing what doesn't. You have total freedom of choice here. Pick and choose from my suggestions, or try them all. It's up to you.

Detoxification of the body is a vast subject. As mentioned earlier, this book is not a comprehensive physical detox guide. And I am not a doctor. This book is just me, a Certified Holistic Health Practitioner and Integrative Nutrition Health Coach, sharing with you some of the things that have worked for me and my clients, family, and friends.

There might be only one suggestion here that you like and that makes a significant difference in your life. Or you might try everything suggested here. Experiment. Be curious. Have fun. Just be sure to consult with a doctor before making any drastic changes or using supplements.

Now, let's dive in.

Keep It Simple

Let's not make this complicated. There is so much advice out there when it comes to detoxing your body, especially in the realm of dietary advice. A lot of it involves supplements and other products. Although I've explored that route personally, for the most part, I prefer to keep things simple and practical—and affordable—especially when it comes to advising others. So that's what I'll share here, the basics:

1. Drink enough water for sufficient hydration and toxin excretion. For extra detox support, add a tablespoon of apple cider vinegar or the juice of half a lemon in the mornings to stimulate your liver. *Brush your teeth after, to protect the enamel!*

2. Reduce or avoid processed foods (for example, white sugar, white flour), alcohol, and products containing artificial ingredients.

3. Focus your diet on whole foods, especially greens and high-fiber foods. Greens help clean your blood, and fiber increases regularity and therefore toxin elimination.

4. Try oil pulling at least a few times a week, if not daily. In addition to removing toxins, it's great for oral hygiene. *What's oil pulling? Keep reading to find out!*

5. Take care of your skin. Exfoliate, such as by dry brushing. Wear breathable clothing. And moisturize with coconut oil instead of body lotion, unless it clogs your pores. *More on body-care products in the Home chapter...*

6. Consider chlorella for gentle, daily detoxing, plus blood sugar balancing. *Consult with a doctor first.*

7. Sweat it out by working out. Even if you don't break a sweat, working out is great for detoxing—not just your body, but also your mind.

8. Get regular, and stay regular. Having healthy bowel

movements is crucial here. And most of what's listed above will help with that.

These are some basic and relatively easy ways to have a healthier, cleaner, clearer body. If you want something more "hard core," or a jump-start that feels like a reset, see the Resources section for more on cleanses. And if you choose a more extensive cleanse or detox protocol, be sure to consult with your doctor and consider working with a certified health coach for support. But first, before exploring a more extreme and possibly pricey option, see if this more gentle and gradual approach works for you after looking more closely at my main suggestions.

What You Drink

Hydration is an essential part of health and an essential part of detoxing, so water yourself as if you were a plant! Drinking enough water is one of the simplest and most fundamental things you can do to improve your overall well-being—body, mind, and spirit. When we are dehydrated, our energy is low, we make poor decisions, and our digestion and elimination systems are impaired.

If you're already well-hydrated, congratulations! This section may not be so necessary for you. But if you're not, consider that even making one change—drinking enough water—can make a huge difference in how you feel.

But what's considered enough? Depends on who you ask. You can aim for that old and familiar standard of eight glasses of water per day. Or you can do the math: various sources now say to forget about the eight glasses a day and instead to drink half your body weight in ounces daily (for example, if you weigh 150 pounds, you'd drink seventy-five ounces of water a day). I've also heard some say to drink a gallon a day, regardless of your weight. However, overhydration *can* occur, so whether you experiment with drinking eight glasses a day, doing the math, or taking other advice, you may want to consult with a physician before making any dramatic adjustments to your water intake.

Although it is possible to overhydrate, dehydration is more common. If you've been dehydrated, it's likely that you'll notice how much better you feel when you start drinking more water, however much that may be. Over time, you'll get a feel for how much water you need, which might also vary depending on things like your weight, your activity level, the climate you're in, and any healing processes you're going through.

Be aware of these signs, which might indicate you are dehydrated:

- Increased thirst
- Dry mouth
- Tired or sleepy
- Decreased urine output
- Urine is low volume and more yellowish than normal
- Headache
- Dry skin
- Dizziness
- Few or no tears
- Bad mood
- Difficulty with decision-making

If drinking enough water feels challenging for you, focus on the benefits, and think about how much better you'll feel. In addition to alleviating the symptoms of dehydration that are listed above, benefits of staying hydrated include:

- More energy

- Better mood
- Clearer mind, enhanced focus, better decision-making
- Less overeating
- Fewer cravings
- Fewer headaches and other aches or pains
- Improved elimination—toxin excretion through urine, and more regularity with better bowel movements

You'll also want to set yourself up for success in practical ways, especially if you're someone who doesn't like water. I've always liked water, but I've had clients who don't. So here are some tips:

How to stay hydrated:

- Have a dedicated water bottle, preferably glass or stainless steel to avoid toxins in plastic. Keep that bottle with you, and refill it as needed.
- Set reminders in your phone if needed, or be old school and use Post-it notes. Some of my clients have used both.
- If it would make drinking more appealing, add positive words or messages to the outside of your bottle. This can also help detox your mind!
- Drink most of your water in the morning and afternoon. Definitely drink some in the evening, too, but not so much that it disrupts your sleep.
- Reward yourself every time you drink some water.
- Use electrolyte tabs or other healthy ways to flavor water (for example, infusions of mint, berries, cucumbers, lemon, etc.).
- Drink herbal tea (non-caffeinated).

- "Eat" your water by consuming more high-water content veggies and fruits, such as cucumbers, watermelon, or celery.

Easy peasy, right? You can do it. And you'll feel better when you do.

Before we move on to what you eat, let's also look at what *not* to drink—or at least what to limit. Whether you cut something out completely or just reduce it totally depends on what the *it* is and on your state of well-being and your goals. For optimal results, I highly recommend completely cutting out these things for a period of time. Then you can reintroduce them little by little and notice how you feel, or just continue to avoid them indefinitely depending upon what's best for you.

Drinks to avoid:

- *Alcohol:* No shame if you like to drink. But in addition to alcohol being a depressant and a diuretic (and therefore dehydrating), large amounts of ethanol is toxic—as in *poisonous*. Our bodies are designed to tolerate and process a certain amount of toxicity, but watch your alcohol intake. For some, moderation may be okay. But for those who are more sensitive to alcohol, cut it out completely or mostly.
- *Soda and other drinks that have sugar or artificial sweeteners added:* Sugar and artificial sweeteners are essential to cut out when detoxing, because sugar depletes the body of essential minerals and also feeds pathogens. And anything artificial is a big *no no* while detoxing—and I'd say even when not detoxing.
- *Milk:* Dairy may not be something you need to cut

out of your diet forever, but it's a good thing to test out, and definitely something to avoid while cleansing or detoxing. Dairy can create inflammation and produce more mucus, even if you're not allergic to it or lactose intolerant. So just give it a rest for at least a few weeks.

- *Coffee and other caffeinated beverages:* Caffeine dehydrates, and while detoxing, you need to stay more hydrated than usual. If you're a caffeine addict, quitting it all cold turkey might be too much to ask of you. In that case, you can just decrease your intake over time, *and* be sure to drink extra water to combat the dehydrating effects.

Yikes! I know that last one might be the hardest. If so, it's definitely your call whether you go completely without or simply reduce—or just focus on cutting the other things out. If you drink coffee daily, cutting it out completely while detoxing in other ways could result in a pretty harsh healing reaction. Whether or not it's worth it depends on your health and your goals. You can also consult with me as a health coach or with another health care provider on what the best approach would be in your situation.

Just know that whenever you cut out things like sugar, alcohol, or caffeine, there can be an unpleasant reaction if you're accustomed to ingesting these things on a regular basis. You may feel worse before feeling better. So remember to keep your eye on the prize, on how you want to feel, on having more energy that's sustainable and not dependent upon a substance.

Another option is to substitute. There are stevia-sweetened or fruit juice–sweetened sodas. And green tea is sometimes suggested as a coffee replacement during detoxes. It still has caffeine, but less, and there are other health benefits to green tea. You can also choose not to cut out caffeine and just focus on the other suggestions. There's no general right or wrong here. It all depends on what your goals are, what you're ready for, what you want. Some of that may be clear from the get go. Some of it may become clearer or shift along the way. You can do this all on your own, or along with an accountability buddy. You might also consider reaching out to me or to another coach for guidance and support.

The key things to remember here are:

- Drink more water, unless you're already sufficiently hydrated (or overhydrated).
- Avoid alcohol, milk, sugary drinks, and caffeinated drinks for maximum detox results and benefits.

What You Eat

You've probably heard the saying "you are what you eat." And it's true. What we eat fuels us. It feeds our cells, it powers us, and it energizes us, but it can also do the opposite. It can gunk up our systems, it can drain our energy, it can even disempower us in the case of food addictions and emotional eating. And, speaking of emotions, food also affects our moods and our thoughts.

When I was a teenager, I was in a nearly fatal car accident. About a year later, when I was seventeen, I felt very depressed. Rather than taking medication, I started reading a book called *Food & Mood*, by Elizabeth Somer, and it made a big difference in how I started thinking and feeling. I learned that some of the emotional toxicity I was feeling came from what I was eating. I learned that dietary detoxes can improve not only our physical well-being, but also our emotional well-being. *Food & Mood* inspired me to change how I was eating, which then changed how I felt—for the better. If you're interested in how your mental or emotional health can be affected by food, I highly recommend that book.

Of course there's something to be said for mind over matter in terms being able to eat and drink whatever you want without any side effects! But there's no denying that what you eat—and avoid eating—is an essential part of detoxing your life, not only due to the physical, but also the mental and emotional effects of what we ingest.

Food—what we eat and how much we eat—can be a touchy subject. In *The Multi-Orgasmic Diet,* I emphasize the importance of *not feeling restricted.* However, sometimes restriction is what we need. It's just important to be ready for it, to not feel like it's punishment, to reframe it. Instead of focusing on feeling *restricted* because of what you are limiting or cutting out completely, focus on feeling good about the healthy choices you make. Mindset is a foundational component of making healthy, sustainable changes. Feeling like these changes are coming from a place of self-love and self-care rather than punishment, or not feeling good enough, makes the changes easier to implement.

Just be honest with yourself. If you feel tired or lethargic after you eat, it's likely that something needs to change. And this isn't about weight or body shape or size. This is about how you feel physically and emotionally. This is about whether or not you have the energy to live the life you want to live. So it's wise to recognize that if you don't feel how you want to feel, if you don't have the energy you want to have, then it could be what you're eating, how much you're eating, or even something like if you're *chewing* thoroughly. It could be the combination of foods you're eating together. It could be from drinking during meals, which can dilute the digestive enzymes, making your body work harder. If you really want to feel your best, you have to be like a detective and commit to figuring out what's sabotaging your success—even if what's sabotaging it is just your mindset and beliefs, which we'll explore in the Mind chapter.

The bottom line here is if your cravings result in choices you know are affecting your physical and/or emotional health, then try using the tips here; you may also want to check out *The Multi-Orgasmic Diet*. For now, though, for the sake of simplicity, start with the general modifications to your diet that can produce a gradual, more natural detox. This advice will also be useful for ongoing maintenance if you choose to do a more extreme jump-start type of cleanse.

Why Avoid Sugar and Refined or Processed Foods?

Sugar can mess with your mood and deplete your body of nutrients. It can also give you dramatic energy spikes followed by dramatic crashes. And it can be addictive. It also suppresses the immune system and feeds candida, which can cause a variety of maladies, including increased infections, thrush, bloating, joint pain, digestive issues, and lethargy. If you believe all that to be true, then it's easy to see why some people say sugar is *toxic*, and that can actually make it easier to cut out completely or at least reduce your intake.

However, be careful here. Be realistic with where you're at. Are you really going to cut out sugar completely? Are you just going to cut out sweets but not read labels or ask at restaurants if sugar is an ingredient, even in savory items? I say *be careful* because it's not good to think of something you're eating as poison or disease-causing unless you're really serious about cutting it out completely and feel the need to use fear as your fuel. Otherwise, you're just making it more harmful by believing it's harmful. If sugar is something you want to eat in moderation, it's important to view it as *non*-toxic when consumed in moderation. And it's important to enjoy the heck out of it! I sure do.

But if you don't know whether or not you need to cut out sugar, I suggest completely avoiding it for thirty days, or at the very least ten days, as an experiment. It can take some time to see how you feel without it in order to then notice any negative effects of eating it again. I believe that unless a medical condition requires you to make a big change here, then it's a very personal choice when it comes to whether or not you're strict about avoiding sugar or allowing it in moderation—if you're not addicted and truly can handle moderation.

As for refined and processed foods, they can clog up your system and be devoid of nutrients and minerals. For example, white rice is actually a remedy for diarrhea; it's constipating— not at all what we want when detoxing. And just like sugar, you decide if you are going to be super strict about this, or every once in a while indulge your taste buds in some refined and processed foods. For example, I sometimes do eat white rice with curry or teriyaki—or when my grandmother would make rice pudding—but other than that, I generally avoid it. If you really want to detox, though, if you want a clean slate, then there does need to be a commitment to total avoidance for at least a short period of time.

I also recommend making a commitment and setting yourself up for success by going through your pantry, fridge, and freezer. Throw stuff away. Feel guilt-free about tossing this stuff out. As I like to say, "Better in the garbage than in your body!" And if you find things you want to toss that haven't been opened and aren't expired, you can donate them. Clean this stuff out to help you avoid temptation and habit, to send a clear message to the universe and to yourself, and to make room for the healthier foods that will be replacing them. If you live with others, get them on board or find a way to compromise and have a designated area for the foods they're still eating that you're avoiding. Ideally that area would be out of sight or out of reach.

Why Eat More Whole Foods, Especially Greens?

Whole foods are nutrient dense and are what your body really yearns for. Cravings arise when your body yearns for missing nutrients. Or cravings can be part of emotional eating, like an attempt to fill a void, soothe pain, feel pleasure, or numb out. When it's nutrients your body is crying out for, eating whole foods will satisfy you and give you the pure and clean energy you need. This can also assist in crowding out the emotional eating types of cravings. By filling up on all the good foods that really nourish your cells, you'll reduce cravings for the things you're better off avoiding.

Whole foods also have more fiber, which will assist you in eliminating waste through regular bowel movements. A combination of sufficient hydration and a high-fiber diet, as well as exercise, is essential for preventing constipation and for encouraging bigger, better bowel movements as part of ongoing detoxification.

As for why I suggest eating more greens? Because chlorophyll supports your body's natural blood-cleansing process. According to Paul Pitchford, author of *Healing with Whole Foods*, the liver, which plays a big role in the processing of toxins, loves two things: a simple diet and greens. So, if you want to detox and make your liver happy, keep it simple, and fill up on greens!

Beware of the Dirty Dozen

Make sure those greens are organic, and consult the current "dirty dozen" list for the twelve types of produce that should always be purchased organic. If you're on a tight budget, it's not necessary for *everything* you buy to be organic. But chemical pesticides and herbicides are toxins that have been linked to various health conditions and birth defects. Therefore, the Environmental Working Group says to watch out for these:

- Strawberries
- Spinach
- Kale
- Nectarines
- Apples
- Grapes
- Peaches
- Cherries
- Pears
- Tomatoes
- Celery
- Potatoes

That's the Dirty Dozen list for the year 2020. Check the Resources section for more on organic food and if you'd like a link to the most up-to-date and downloadable version of the Dirty Dozen list as well as a list of the Clean Fifteen—the fifteen fruits and veggies that have the lowest concentration of pesticides and therefore are considered safe even if purchasing conventional instead of organic.

What Else?

We've covered some basic, foundational ways you can detox on the physical level. If you want more, here are the other things I suggested at the beginning of the chapter:

Coconut oil for moisturizing and oil pulling: I recommend coconut oil as a natural moisturizer, but more on that in the Home chapter. Here I want to share about oil pulling, which is an Ayurvedic practice traditionally done with sesame oil. Feel free to use coconut oil instead.

Place one tablespoon of oil (or less at first, while getting used to it) in your mouth and continuously "pull" it through your teeth for twenty minutes (or ten minutes to start). The "pulling" is not just like swishing around mouthwash. You want to feel like you're pulling the oil through your teeth. This pulls toxins and bacteria out of your gums and salivary glands. When your timer goes off, spit it out—but not down the sink! I use a bag that I keep in my freezer; when the bag is full, it goes into the garbage.

Dry skin brushing: Purchase a brush that is specifically for this purpose, or you can use a loofah or rough washcloth instead. Before showering, brush your body, stroking towards the heart. Although the primary benefit of dry skin brushing is exfoliation, you may also be assisting your body's natural detoxification processes by stimulating the circulatory and lymphatic systems. Some say do this daily, but others say that can be damaging to your skin. So I'm just recommending once or twice a week, to be safe. You can do some research or talk to a healthcare professional if you're curious about doing it more often.

Chlorella: Chlorella is a supplement that assists in gently detoxing your body. It also regulates blood sugar, which is extra supportive when modifying your diet. It's high in iodine and vitamin K, though, so please be sure to consult with your doctor before adding supplements like this to your diet, especially if you're taking blood thinning medications or if you have been diagnosed with—or suspect you might have—*any* type of thyroid condition.

Sweat: You can sweat out toxins by working out or by using a sauna. Even working out without breaking a sweat is great for detoxing because it gets your blood pumping, and it's good for your emotional well-being. Wearing breathable clothing is also beneficial.

Letting Go of the Crap We Carry

In addition to sweating them out, there's another way we get rid of toxins that needs to be addressed here, as it's a big part of being healthy in body, mind, and spirit. And that is... poop. We all do it. And in order to detox your life, you'll need to make sure you're having regular, healthy bowel movements, since it's one primary way we excrete toxins.

As mentioned above, in addition to drinking enough water, eating whole foods high in fiber, and getting regular exercise will help prevent constipation. If you need a little extra assistance in the regularity department, please avoid stimulant laxatives. There are natural options, such as eating prunes, dates, or dried goldenberries before bed. Ground flaxseed in warm water is also an option.

Although there are mixed opinions out there about the ideal frequency of bowel movements, the main question is: are you regularly (daily) eliminating a sufficient amount of waste? To fully address colon health and troubleshoot both constipation and diarrhea would go beyond the scope of this book, so here we will just take a brief look at constipation.

Some reasons for constipation include:

- Dehydration
- Constipating foods
- Lack of fiber
- Stress and anxiety
- Trauma

Some solutions for constipation include:

- Drinking more water throughout the day

- Eating dried goldenberries, prunes, or dates before bed
- Drinking flax tea before bed
- Abdominal massage
- Acupuncture and acupressure points
- Herbs
- Aloe vera juice
- Exercise, even just walking
- Shaking (gently shaking the body or using a rebounder to bounce)
- Meditation and qigong
- Psychotherapy if there are psychological barriers
- Colon cleanse with proper instructions, products, and guidance

If you're experiencing constipation, and implementing the suggestions from the previous sections of this chapter don't make a difference, you can explore some of the additional solutions listed above. I won't go through each one here, but as a former massage therapist, I do want to say something about abdominal massage.

If you'd like to try it yourself, the most basic way is to gently rub your belly in a clockwise motion—following the ascending colon up on the right, and the descending colon down on the left. This can be done directly on the skin with or without lotion or oil, or it can be done over clothing. If you have the time and money to see a professional who practices Mayan abdominal massage, you can go to a session or two and receive instructions on self-care massage to continue on your own. Chi Nei Tsang is also a form of professional abdominal massage.

If your bowel movements are regular, this may not be a priority to add into your routine, but it's still beneficial. However, if you experience constipation, I highly recommend abdominal massage, whether from a professional or from yourself. And I highly recommend you do whatever it takes to get regular—and stay regular—because letting go of both the physical and metaphorical crap you carry is essential for detoxing your life.

Final Thoughts on the Body

Although there are plenty of fad diets and detoxes and cleanses out there, what we've looked at in this chapter are some simple things you can do to get your body feeling cleaner and clearer —and to keep it feeling good. Depending on your needs, challenges, and goals, you might choose to be strict about the suggestions above. Or you might adopt an 80/20 rule, either in general or after a detox. For example, maybe after cutting out sugar and processed foods for thirty days, you decide 80 percent of your diet will be whole foods and sugar-free, but 20 percent will be whatever the heck you want it to be.

Decide for yourself what works best for you. It may take some trial and error. But you can do it. And when you clean out the body and do your best to keep it detoxified? Your mind and emotions will be clearer too. But there's probably still more to do. And since what you put *on* your body—and what you breathe into your body—are also relevant, we'll look at things like body-care and cleaning products in the Home chapter. But first, in the Mind chapter, you'll receive guidance on how to clean up and clear out toxic, self-limiting thoughts and beliefs.

If you're having a hard time with the body detoxing, or feel you've already got that covered and don't need to implement any suggestions from this chapter, the mental detox is a good alternative starting point. Or if you're ready to move forward with detoxing your body before finishing the book, you can use the Sample Plan book bonuses to support you in the process: www.rebeccacliogould.com/detoxbonuses.

MIND

ALTHOUGH WE STARTED with the body as a foundation, the mind is just as important, if not more so. In fact, some would say start with your mind when detoxing your life. And that's certainly an option. I find that it all overlaps. And sometimes physically cleaning out the body is a great way to get more in alignment with cleaning up and clearing out the mind. For others, starting with the mind makes more sense. Or perhaps the very best is to approach them simultaneously.

One benefit of this book being short is that you can read through the whole thing before *really* getting started, and then you can dive back in with the specifics when you're ready. Or you can do what I call *layering*. In my first book, *The Multi-Orgasmic Diet*, I shared over eighty practices for cultivating sexual energy and awakening sensuality to help women fill up on the pleasure and pulse of life in order to feel more fulfilled —and therefore make healthier choices more naturally. Because it can feel overwhelming to take on so many new activities all at once, I suggested layering, which is also an option here. It just means that you start with one thing, maybe two, and then as you feel like you've gotten into a groove with that and are ready to add more, you add another thing into the mix.

And there's no need to eventually be doing it *all.* Just add whichever suggestions or practices you like, whenever it works best for you. This way you are making changes at a pace that is comfortable and sustainable, which will prevent burnout and overwhelm. I want to set you up for success rather than for failure; I don't want you to quit before you have a chance to see the wonders that can be worked here.

And one of the wonders of working the *Detox Your Life* system? A cleaner and clearer mind. A mind that is more pure, more optimistic, more solution-oriented. Uncluttered. Unburdened. Open. Free. And in order to detox your life, it is *crucial* to detox your mind.

Our minds are powerful. And you can put your mind to good use, for your betterment. But you can also use your mind to sabotage and harm—usually without being aware that that's what you're doing.

Oftentimes, our minds get gunked up without us even realizing it. Things your loved ones say, things strangers say, the news, social media, TV shows and movies—they work their way into your subconscious and influence your thoughts and feelings, and therefore your life!

A lot of the programming occurs when we're children. Yes, programming. You see, the brain is like a computer. There's all this input going in, all this programming, and that affects how we operate in the world and what we put out into the world. Our thoughts create our beliefs. And our beliefs result in our actions, which create our lived experiences (aka, *life*).

So, if how you think creates your life, then you can change your life by changing your thinking. Sounds good, right? But oftentimes it's easier said than done. It's certainly possible, but requires conscious awareness, *subconscious* reprogramming, and commitment to making deliberate choices that support

your intentions. It requires new thoughts for creating the
programs you want to run.

What You Think

What you think has power. Those thoughts become your
beliefs. And your beliefs dictate your choices, your actions,
your experiences, and therefore your life. This is worthy of
repeating because it is so important. And it's important to look
at how our toxic thoughts can get in the way of us feeling our
best and having the experiences we truly want for ourselves.
Just think about it for a moment.

Do you ever find yourself thinking negative thoughts about
someone or something? Of course! That's human. Or how
about beating yourself up over something? Or thinking about
how *hard* things are or that you *just can't* do something? How
much of your thinking consists of judgment, complaints, or
doubt? And is your mind too busy or overcrowded with useless
stories and thoughts spinning in your head?

Imagine how good it would feel to have a quieter and
kinder mind. A mind that is your best friend, your biggest fan,
and your wisest mentor? This is possible for you.

We all have negative thought patterns and emotions from
time to time. Sometimes we truly are our own worst enemy.
Our self-limiting beliefs can sabotage our happiness and the
fulfillment of our dreams. But there's something we can do.
There's something you can do.

You can become consciously aware of what's happening in
that head of yours. You can view your brain like a computer,
delete the corrupt files, wipe out the viruses, and run new
programs. You can upgrade your belief systems by consciously
choosing your thoughts and reprogramming your subconscious mind.

Here's the catch though: you can't just go through the

motions of thinking differently. Although at first you may have to "fake it till you make it," those new thoughts need to turn into new beliefs. For best results, you have to enter into a deeply relaxed state, such as through meditation, to get beyond the conscious mind and into the subconscious mind. And you have to truly believe—truly *feel*—what you are thinking, in order for it to be effective and sustainable.

How to do this? Keep reading.

Think a New Thought

You can "crowd out" the toxic thinking with new thoughts, with positive self-talk, affirmations, and intentions. You can spend time visualizing, consciously daydreaming, and feeling into the imagined reality you want to manifest.

You can reprogram your mind to be as clean and clear and loving as you want by filling your mind so full of healing, positive, loving thoughts that there's no room—or less room—for the harmful thoughts. And using guided meditations, hypnosis, or listening to a recording of yourself reciting affirmations as you fall asleep can get them into your subconscious.

You're welcome to skip over the following practice of identifying toxic thoughts and just go straight to focusing on what you want. However, it might be beneficial to learn how to identify and catch harmful thought patterns to help you break the habit of thinking those thoughts. You'll also learn more about how to transform them. Our most negative thoughts can be like messengers, signaling us to what needs healing within. So let's give them some attention instead of just trying to sweep them under the rug.

ACTIVITY:
THINK A NEW THOUGHT—WITH FEELING!

1. Take inventory.

Set aside some quiet, uninterrupted time for this. Get out a notebook or journal, or whatever you use to take notes, and have it near you. Sit comfortably, relax your body, and write down the thought patterns you know you already have that don't feel good. (*For example, Nothing ever works out for me. I can't figure it out. Others can't be trusted. I have to do it all myself. Nobody understands me, etcetera.*)

Think about things you often say internally or out loud, the things that are excuses. The things that make you feel stuck or small. The "I don't know's" and the "but I can't, because's." The "I would if I could, but's." The regrets. The self-flagellations. The self-criticism. The self-doubt. The fears. The complaints and judgments about self, others, and the world.

Drawing a blank when trying to come up with your list? Feeling blocked? Reading through your journals—or even old emails or social media posts—can reveal patterns and help you identify some harmful, limiting beliefs you have about yourself, about others, about life.

Note: There may be no need to dig all of that up. You can just start paying attention in your current daily life, or you can take more time to dig deep into past patterns. It's up to you.

As you go throughout your days, your weeks, your life, take note of any toxic thoughts that arise—any thoughts that feel icky, that bring you down, that aren't kind to yourself or to others. Jot them down to deal with later or start flipping the script immediately.

2. Flip the scripts.

This is the fun part, but it does require that you have written something down to work with—or you can do it in your head in the moment of identifying the thought.

With each thought or belief you identified as harmful, toxic, negative, or limiting, rewrite it as something that would feel better. Sometimes this will be an opposite statement, such as going from "I'm such an idiot" to "I am an intelligent being, and I know what's best for me."

Other times it will not be so straightforward. For example, it might be going from "I'm such an idiot" to "I'm learning to have better discernment," or "Everything is working out just how it's supposed to. And I'm learning and growing from this." It really depends on you and where you're at and what feels best. Maybe going from "I'm such an idiot" to "I'm intelligent and wise and always make the best choices for myself," will work for you.

Experiment. Play. Anything will be a step up, an improvement. And for it to really create a shift, you need to be able to really feel it and receive it as true; that's why sometimes the extreme opposites won't always work, unless you can get into the *feeling* state of it. If you're a spiritual person, or would like to develop your spirituality, this is a great opportunity to practice recognizing and affirming the Truth of who you are as a Divine being who really is perfect and whole, always and in all ways. And if you're not into spirituality, you can ignore that last sentence.

Whichever statements you choose, practice repeating them like affirmations, before going to sleep and/or when you wake up in the morning, since that is when your subconscious mind is most easily programmed.

Some people also like creating sticky notes and placing them around their home. You can also text yourself these statements or set reminders or alarms in your phone so that they pop up from time to time. You can record yourself saying them and then listen to the recording before sleep, when you wake up, or any time you need a little reminder.

One practice I love is taking my own kind of "power walk"—a power of the mind walk, during which I recite an affirmation or prayer over and over again during the walk. Remember, it's gotta be with feeling, real feeling. You need to really feel it. And in this case, it's okay to try out faking it until you make it. Sometimes that works. And if it doesn't, then the language of the affirmation or prayer may need some tweaking.

Give this time. Be patient with yourself. When we've spent years thinking a certain way, it can be hard to change. And although sustainable dramatic transformations are possible, recognize that it might instead be subtle shifts over time, through a lifetime practice of just being more self-aware and catching yourself in those negative, limiting thoughts, and then course-correcting in the moment or shortly thereafter. Just doing your best. Day by day. Moment by moment. Focusing on progress, not perfection.

You will notice positive shifts in your life if you commit to this process. You'll feel lighter and brighter. You'll feel more joy and enjoyment. More contentment. And the choices you make, the things you do and say, will reflect this cleaner and clearer mind.

What You Say

Our words, the ones we speak out loud, also have power. Words can create or destroy our dreams, our relationships, our happiness. And they can either support or harm others. To do less harm, ask yourself if your words are kind, necessary, and true— the triple filter or three gates test recommended by Socrates, as well as Buddhists and other teachers. What a wonderful thing to ask yourself before speaking—you can also use it when evaluating your thoughts!

Another valuable question comes from Don Miguel Ruiz's *The Four Agreements*: are you impeccable with your word, or do you spew venom with your tongue?

What we say silently will also be considered here. And I'm

not talking about thoughts in general. We explored that in the previous section. I'm talking about the imaginary conversations —or monologues or diatribes—we run in our head before or instead of talking to someone when there's conflict to resolve.

I must admit I've said some pretty venomous things to those who have hurt me—not out loud, but in my head. Usually it comes up like this uncontrollable spontaneous thing out of the blue. *That stupid &#@$^! What an @$$#*!%.* I'll spare you the details, but you get the point. Sometimes it's therapeutic to vent, such as by writing out or speaking out loud all of the yuckiness to help work out anger, hurt, and other uncomfortable emotions. But in order to get to a place of peace—and perhaps even gratitude—there's gotta be some intentionality and awareness about the process. This comes up in the Relationships chapter too.

There's so much growth and learning that can happen when we become more self-aware and can observe the negative thoughts and words without attaching truth to them. Be as objective as possible when observing your own mind. Look deeper at what it's telling you. What's unresolved? What pain needs tending to?

Asking these questions and answering them can be difficult, but it's worth the payoff. You can also see if it works for you to bypass this type of intensive self-inquiry by using "shortcuts" such as crowding out negative words and thoughts with positive affirmations or listening to guided meditations.

The thing to recognize is that when we speak in an unkind or otherwise harmful way, it's coming from some fear-based part of ourselves—and it's not really true. It's not the "capital T Truth" of who we really are. It's just some part of ourselves that has separated from love, compassion, humility, humanity, oneness. And we can tap back into the higher Truth of who we are with practices such as Sheng Zhen, and other forms of meditation—or even just through journaling, taking a walk in nature, or laughing with a friend.

The more we work on cleaning up our thoughts and clearing our minds, the more our words will follow. Our words will be more kind, necessary, and true.

Warning: it's common for people to bond through commiserating and complaining. As you detox your mind and become more self-aware, there may be certain people or conversations that no longer resonate with you. This can feel really uncomfortable and perhaps even confusing.

What will you do? Will you join in and match their tone and go down a rabbit hole of negativity? Will you stay rooted in yourself and therefore possibly elevate the tone by reframing things? Will you empathize and join in for a little while but then politely change the subject to prevent going down that rabbit hole?

As you increase your self-awareness and start thinking more positively, as you clean and clear your own energy, your body, and your mind, you just might naturally decrease the prevalence of people trying to complain around you or commiserate with you. Or you might get better at holding space for others without getting brought down by their troubles.

Just watch out for spiritual bypassing and lack of true empathy. As you begin to elevate your thoughts and words, it may feel challenging to be supportive when loved ones are sharing their pain with you. I must admit that my own desire to not get entangled with other people's painful stories or complaining has sometimes resulted in me not being a good listener or a good friend. Sometimes people just need to be heard. If it's hard for you to just listen, because it feels harmful, you can ask if they want help with a solution. You can try to redirect the conversation. But giving unsolicited advice or trying to get them to shift their attitude may not be the best move to make. That being said, if trying to just listen to whatever they're saying is bringing you down, it's also necessary for you to have healthy boundaries, which we will look at more in the Relationships chapter. Now it's time for our "power of words" activity!

ACTIVITY:
THE WORDS WE USE AND THE POWER OF WORDS

Words have power, especially if you're a sensitive person. If you journal, you can review your journaling to identify words or phrases that come up a lot and that reinforce negative feelings or self-limiting beliefs. Or maybe you noticed that in the previous practice. And in your conversations with people—or even with yourself—start heightening your awareness of the words you use. You can also listen for this in what others are saying and writing.

Be on the lookout for words and phrases such as the following:

I don't know. I used to say this a lot. "I don't know." "I just don't know." "I don't really know." Although not knowing can be a good thing, even a freeing thing, alternatively it can indicate self-doubt and have a negative tone. It also can be an avoidance mechanism—a way to deflect.

Depending on why these words are coming up, you can either start replacing them with statements like "I know what's best for me," "I'm figuring it out," or "Let me sit with this and get back to you." Or, if you really *don't know*, then you can try *embracing* not knowing as a good thing; this, of course, like many things, may depend on context.

Never. Never is a very definitive word, a word that limits possibility. "Things never work out for me." "I never get my way." "He/She/They never..." "It's/I'm never good enough."

First of all, is it really true, this "never"? Usually, "never" is an exaggeration. But even if it's not, it's worth looking at how to shift the thinking and language to open up for more possibility. Limiting possibility by having a "never" type of mentality can be quite harmful. A detoxed mind is an open mind—open to limitless possibilities.

Can't. There's a difference between *can't* and *won't.* There's a difference of choice and perspective. And what's written above about possibilities also comes into play here. As we begin to detox the mind, we feel more capable, like there's more we *can* do. More we can choose to do. And most importantly, that we have a choice over what we can and can't do, what we will and won't do.

Should. Have you ever heard someone say "stop shoulding on yourself"? This word implies an obligation, a sense of pressure, and not an authentic desire. However, it's also so commonly used that it doesn't necessarily always indicate inauthenticity. It's not always to be interpreted as a command to do something you don't really want to do. That being said, when you notice a *should* bubbling up in or out of you, take a moment to examine what's really going on to see if there's a better way to express yourself.

For example, does "I should practice yoga more" really mean "I feel better when I practice yoga, so I want to make more time for it" or does it mean "I don't really like yoga but people keep telling me to try it, so I feel pressure"? And does "we should hang out" mean "I want to spend time with you; let's make a plan!" or does it mean "I don't really want to hang out with you but think you want me to want to hang out with you"?

Get curious about what's really going on when a *should* arises, and then adjust your language accordingly.

It's so hard. Okay, yes, sometimes things feel hard, sometimes things *are* hard, and it's okay to acknowledge that. But sometimes we make things even harder—or harder for longer

—by getting stuck in a tape loop of this thought and perception of something being hard. My favorite remedy for this is actually an Easy button from Staples—or more than one! I have one in my house and one in my car, and it totally makes a difference.

What's an Easy button? It's a big red button with the word "Easy" on it, and when you press it, you'll hear a voice say, "That was easy!" And one of the best times to use it is actually after something that wasn't so easy, because it can make you laugh and lighten the mood. You can get one from Staples or through Amazon.

Even if you just decrease or eliminate from your usage the preceding list of words and phrases, without finding any others, that's an awesome detox right there. Your language and your mind will be cleaner and clearer when you reduce or completely avoid words and phrases that keep you stuck or bring you down rather than uplifting you or at least bringing you into a place of neutrality. Remember to check your words (and your thoughts!) with those three gates:

Is it kind?
Is it necessary?
Is it true?

Asking these questions will help you course-correct if you're headed down a toxic path. I've certainly caught myself before hitting the send button on more than one email or text message, thanks to those three questions. Sometimes it's better to just take a breath. Delete that message, or stop yourself from saying what you're thinking about saying, and whittle it down to what's kind, necessary, and true.

A big part of detoxing your mind is increasing your self-awareness enough to catch any "stinkin' thinkin'" and then to replace it with something better. That's what you can do for yourself when it's your own thoughts and words showing signs of toxicity. But what about when it's coming from other sources? Let's take a look at that next.

Social Media and News Detox

Because words are powerful and affect our thoughts, which affect our beliefs, we need to take a moment to talk about social media and the news. If you're one of those rare breeds who isn't using social media *or* watching any news, you can skip this section or just skim it. Otherwise, read on...

Social media has become an addiction or habit for many. It's easy to get hooked on checking social media more than just once, twice, or a few times a day. And even if you only check it once or twice, it can still take a toll.

Although social media can be a fun way to connect with others, promote the work you do, find events, and participate in groups, it can also clutter our minds, waste our time, and negatively affect our mental and emotional well-being.

First of all, when you're scrolling through and see things people post that are negative, disturbing, or otherwise triggering, it can adversely affect you even if you think you are desensitized to it. There's also the reward system that gets activated by things like notifications and people liking and commenting on your stuff. This can create an addiction. And then there's the other side of that: feeling bad when it's just crickets.

Hello? Anybody out there??

Clearly, social media can impact our mood in a good way, but it can also create or contribute to stress, anxiety, and depression. I'm not going to ask you to give up on social media altogether, although that's certainly an option. What I am asking is that you consider decreasing your usage, and start by taking a complete break.

Choose an amount of time for a total break: a week, or a month? Somewhere in between? If it has truly become an addiction or habit, giving it up for at least four weeks is best. If you're not willing to give it up completely, you can set boundaries and guidelines instead. For example, only checking it a certain number of times a day and only at designated times or windows of time. There's a lot of leeway here depending on what you need, but be truthful with yourself about what you think would work best. I encourage you to try the more extreme detox here.

As for the news, yes, we need to be informed about what's happening in the world. But there are a variety of ways to get the news. Reading only the headlines might be the best when doing a news detox, if not quitting completely. It may still feel like a downer to read the headlines, especially if they're "click bait" headlines, but without the details of the whole story, sometimes it's easier to let it go; you can feel informed without going down a rabbit hole or feeling consumed by the news.

There's also the option of taking in the news with a dose of humor. My favorite method of staying informed in a way that's palatable to a sensitive soul like me is the late night shows, such as *The Daily Show*, because, for me, humor counteracts at least some of the toxicity. Laughter is medicine.

Also consider the frequency and time of day that you take in the news—as well as social media newsfeeds that might contain unpleasant messaging. I suggest this *not* be how you start or end the day—not right when you wake up, and not right before bed, because these are times when our subconscious minds are most easily programmed. Use these times of day for healthy, happy-making activities and for taking in positive information and messaging.

How to have a successful media detox:

- Remove the apps from your phone.
- Consider changing your password to something

more complicated and logging out each time so that if you're tempted to cheat, you have to take a moment to consider if you really are going to break the promise you made to yourself.

- Select the amount of time for total avoidance if taking that route (recommended!).
- Select the number of times and the actual time of day you will check your social media accounts and/or the news.
- Keep in mind there's an adjustment period if you're truly addicted to checking these apps and sites. You'll notice yourself going to them without even realizing what you're doing. That's okay. That's why I recommend signing out and changing your password. Make it harder to continue the habit!
- Think back to what it was like, if you're old enough, to when we didn't have these social media apps or the news so readily available on our phones. Find other ways to connect with others, such as FaceTime, Marco Polo, or good ol' phone calls. Find other ways to stimulate your brain and to express yourself, such as journaling, writing a letter, or drawing. Or take more time to just be—to meditate, to go outside, to look around. Social media and news consumption can take a big toll on your energy, mood, and time. Reclaim it!

I took my own advice here and stayed off of Facebook and Instagram for a little over a month while finishing up writing this book. During the first week, I found myself habitually starting to type "facebook" into the internet browser, but since I was logged out, it didn't matter. And soon the habit was broken. *Hooray!*

During my social media break, I felt more at peace and less

anxious, and I felt way more focused and creative. As I re-entered social media after thirty-four days away, I felt hesitant about being back and more mindful of how I want to engage with these platforms. Why? Because I noticed a positive differ-ence in both my mental health and my creative productivity when not using Facebook or Instagram.

Whether you need to quit cold turkey or can find a happy medium, I encourage you to experiment with taking a break from social media, the news, or certain TV shows. Doing so will enable you to enjoy your life more without looking at your screen so much—and without letting other people's words clutter and influence your mind.

Song Lyrics and Music

Speaking of things that influence your mind, music is one of the most powerful ways to influence your mind—to program it, even. Think about how many song lyrics you know by heart, even if you only remember them when you hear the song. Those words are in your subconscious. Music you listen to, especially frequently, can have a big influence on your mood, your thoughts, your beliefs, the words you choose, your vibe—your life! And let's face it: a lot of song lyrics aren't so good for us.

Some are neutral. Some are uplifting. But some are down-right toxic and can adversely influence you subconsciously. Even music that doesn't have lyrics might affect your mood based on the mood of the music. I'm all for using music for catharsis, but there's conscious intention with that. It's like jour-naling or venting. Sometimes you just gotta wallow in it or get it all out of your system—or both. The issue is when it's subcon-sciously affecting you—influencing your thoughts and feelings with things like sad, angry, misogynistic, or codependent lyrics.

MIND   47

Don't get me wrong; some of my favorite songs have the type of lyrics that make me wish I didn't understand English! Some of the crassest songs move me to dance or make me laugh. And I know everyone has different levels of sensitivity and suggestibility. So I'm not asking you to give up listening to your favorite music. Just be mindful about it. And consider adding some more music with positive lyrics if that's not already part of your playlist.

ACTIVITY:
MINDFUL LISTENING AND MUSIC CLEANSE

Mindful listening: Depending on the type of music you listen to, this may not apply. But listen to the lyrics closely, and notice if there are any negative messages in the lyrics or if the music itself feels negative or has a downward spiral or heaviness to it. If you're not sensitive to this type of thing, that's fine. It may be hard to detect.

And there's certainly nothing wrong with enjoying some melancholy music from time to time—as long as it's not having a negative impact on your general vibe and feelings. Sometimes melancholy or angry music feels good. Sometimes it's necessarily cathartic. Just notice how you feel and see if the music you listen to affects your emotions and thoughts in a positive, negative, or neutral way.

Music cleanse: For a minimum of one week, only listen to music without lyrics or with neutral or positive lyrics. If no lyrics, the music itself should have an uplifting or neutral feel to it. If you want to try the cleanse for more than a week, go for ten days or up to thirty days. I believe all it takes is seven to ten days to notice a difference. What difference? Go back to listening to some music you'd listened to before and see if you still like it, or just notice if you've felt more positive or clear-headed while on the music cleanse.

The above practice was inspired by an example from my own life. In the summer of 2008, I was driving to the airport on my way to a Sheng Zhen teacher training. I was listening to Ice Cube really loudly in my car. When I returned home from two weeks of heart-opening meditation and qigong, and not really listening to any music at all, I got in my car, and that type of rap music just didn't resonate anymore. I didn't like it. After some months, I was able to enjoy it again from time to time, but it was pretty amazing just how much I didn't like it right after the combo of a music detox and a couple weeks of mindfulness, meditation, and qigong!

As I already said, your level of sensitivity and suggestibility will play a role in how impactful music is when it comes to your well-being. And our taste in music is very personal. It's okay to like what you like and to dislike what you dislike. But give that practice a try. See what happens. And for some positive music suggestions, check out my Detox Your Life song list in the bonus material.

When in Doubt, Meditate

If you already have a meditation practice, awesome. If you don't, and you truly want to detox your life, it's time to start. It's one of the best ways to detox your mind—to clean and clear it, to reprogram it.

If meditation is hard for you, you can begin with a short amount of time. You can start just by taking a minute or two to notice your breath at multiple times throughout your day. You can also explore various types of meditation. There are plenty of guided meditations and visualizations on YouTube. There are also meditative practices other than just sitting. You can meditate while you walk. You can learn tai chi or qigong, which are like meditations in motion. You can find a class near you, videos online, or join one of my online classes. I've also included a couple of guided meditations for you in the bonus material and provided reading and video recommendations in the Resources section.

And now that you've considered various ways to detox your body and your mind? It's time to look at detoxing your home, your physical environment. Sometimes it's actually easiest to start with the home. It's a good place to practice discernment about what stays and what goes. It's a good place to start reframing how we think and feel about things. And it's important to get some practice detoxing our relationships with the *material* world before diving in to the complex realm of detoxing our relationships with other people! So, up next? Home...

HOME

THE MATERIAL WORLD is full of actual toxins, like fumes and chemicals. And a healthy body can process a lot of that out without experiencing harm. But another way—perhaps a more subtle way—in which the material world can create toxicity? Clutter.

Although we'll touch upon things like air quality and the ingredients found in body-care and cleaning products in this chapter, I'd like to start off with a focus on clutter. In the previous chapter, we looked at how to clear the clutter in your mind, such as through meditation. But you can't just meditate away the physical clutter in your environment. Material clutter and excess block energy flow and therefore can create stagnation in your life, negative emotions, and a sense of overwhelm or confusion. And perhaps you've heard of feng shui? I am not a feng shui consultant, and there's more to it than re-arranging furniture and cleaning up clutter. But one of the main principles is about energy flow.

When energy flow is blocked, there's stagnation, and that can create a toxic environment—whether we're talking about the body or the home you live in. And just like the body needs to be excreting toxins on a daily basis, as well as limiting the intake of toxins, we also benefit from detoxing—and decluttering—our home.

Your environment also contributes to supporting you in continuing habits—whether good or bad. So what you choose to have in your space, and where you place it or how you use it, can also make it easier or harder for you to detox your life. For example, if you watch the news in your bed at night but want to do a news detox, maybe you'll choose to move your TV to another room or even put it in the closet for a while.

Some of what we'll look at in this chapter also applies to your office or work environment if you work outside of your home. For the sake of simplicity, I will primarily be referring to your home, but apply what you can to other places you spend a lot of time in. Some of it will be out of your control, but do what you can. For example, if you work in an office space with others, you can declutter and rearrange *your own* office, cubicle, or desk.

And if there are cleaning products being used that are toxic? Consider putting in a request to management or HR asking if there's any possibility of using different products. It can't hurt to ask. And having some plants around, if permissible depending on where you work, can also improve the energy of your space. Obviously, this won't apply to all work environments. So take what does apply and leave the rest. Focus on the space, or spaces, in which you have a choice and can make healthy modifications.

Just keep in mind the *power* of your mind—if you work somewhere that has some toxins, as in actual poisonous chemicals or a "toxic" atmosphere, do your best to focus on the positives instead of fixating on something potentially harmful. We don't always have total control over our external environment, such as when it's shared with others. And we certainly cannot control other people. But, as we explored in the previous chapter, what we can control is our own thoughts and what we choose to focus on. It could be more harmful to fixate on the things that are toxic and will not be changing than to just accept them and focus more of your thoughts on all that is healthy, all that is good, all that you can do to feel your best.

By focusing on the positive aspects, the harmful ones have less power over you. And doing what you can in terms of diet and other self-care practices can prevent or diminish any possible harmful impact of your external environment. The Energy Egg practice in the Relationship chapter may be useful here too. But first let's talk a bit more about energy.

The Energy of Stuff

Physical possessions have energy. It's not vital life force energy (qi), but it can affect your qi—and therefore your energy level, mood, and overall sense of well-being. For example, if you have a piece of artwork someone gave you, but you had a falling out with that person, then maybe it's best not to have that constant reminder on your wall anymore. Alternatively, you might choose to implement the power of your mind by using affirmations, visualizations, or prayer to cleanse and shift the energy and your associations with this item—it could become an uplifting reminder of the good times or what you've learned and how you've grown since then.

Another example is that practitioners of feng shui avoid dried flowers, as they're believed to represent death. If you really want to keep some dried flowers, such as part of a bridal bouquet, consider pressing them or creating potpourri. Or you could just choose to decide that this knowledge of feng shui's interpretation is not going to affect you. *Mind over matter!* You don't need to let material things, or beliefs about them, have power over you. Even if you still decide to throw them away, you can do so from a cleaner and clearer place rather than from fear or any other negative association.

How Things Make You Feel

Speaking of negative associations, as alluded to above, things have energy in terms of how they make you feel. I already shared a couple of examples, such as artwork or dried flowers, but give it some more thought. Do you have things at home that brighten your day and make you feel good? Do you have things at home that make you feel bad? Guilty? Not good enough? Lonely? Resentful?

Is there a guitar sitting in the corner just gathering dust? Something you never play but feel like you *should*? Is there clothing that you want to fit into but don't? How long have you been holding on to it? Does it make you feel like you're not in the body you want to be in? Do you feel like a failure or not good enough or like there's something wrong with you? Do you have jewelry or some other gift from an ex, and seeing it reminds you of something negative or stirs up feelings of heartbreak or failure or loneliness?

These are just a few examples. Consider getting rid of this type of stuff. If it has sentimental value or you really truly do see yourself using it again someday, then put it somewhere out of sight, or work on the mental detoxing so that you feel good when you see it, excited about the future or filled with joy over the memories.

Our pasts, our memories, can be a wonderful contribution to who we are now. But there can also be stagnation and toxicity when we hold on to things with memories that don't serve us. And although you can try to use mind over matter to shift the energy or association, you can also just get rid of those material possessions.

Whether there are memories attached to it or not, when

you look at something in your home or work environment, notice how it makes you feel. Does it light you up? Bring you down? Or is it neutral? I haven't read her book or watched her show, but I've heard about Marie Kondo and her question: "Does it spark joy?" For years I'd already been asking this in another way, thanks to Laura Lavigne's "Lighten Up!" class in which she teaches you to ask the question: "Is it actively used or deeply cherished?"

One reason why Kondo's and Lavigne's questions are so helpful is that sometimes negative emotions or the toxic impact of some *thing* is subtle. But what's not so subtle is the answer to the questions, "Does it spark joy?" or "Is this deeply cherished or actively used?" These questions tend to be easier to answer. They also get you to focus more on the positive—and then you can just let go of the rest.

The idea here is that you will feel your best when everything in your environment is something that you're happy to have, whether for sentimental reasons or utilitarian ones. And as Laura Lavigne teaches, because each material item is something you are responsible for, you need to ask yourself if it's deserving of your physical space and your mental attention. Is it deserving of your time, energy, and care? If not, say goodbye.

How to Declutter

Now, let's get down to the real nitty gritty of how to detox your space by decluttering. Some of this has already been mentioned above, but here's your cheat sheet, plus some additional tips:

1. Break it down into manageable amounts of time and/or spaces. For example, commit to one closet, or one room, or two out of five drawers. There's no right or wrong in terms of how much or how little to do. Laura Lavigne suggests no more than ninety minutes at a time.

Some people can joyfully handle spending a few hours on decluttering, or making a whole day of it. Some people feel best doing little bits at a time. What you want is to feel a good sense of completion after your decluttering sessions and to not get burned out by them. So select the amount of time and space you can complete while enjoying the process.

2. Sometimes you may just see what it is that needs to be removed. But another option is to take everything out. Let's use clothes in a closet, for example. Take everything out of your closet, and then decide what goes back in. But first? Clean the closet.

3. I like using Laura Lavigne's "actively used or deeply cherished" mantra as a guideline. Try that out for yourself. And please note that "actively used" doesn't necessarily mean *frequently* used; it could be something you use once a year, or even less, like an extension cord or first aid kit. She defines it as something that partners with you to create the life you want. Maybe you don't want a life that requires you to go shopping for an extension cord—or ask to borrow one from someone— on the rare occasion you need one. Maybe you want a life in which you're already prepared! But if you have more than one and really only need one? Give away the extras.

Sometimes it's not about getting rid of something completely, but reducing the amount if you have excess. For things that you don't use often, such as certain types of tools, consider looking into if there's a neighborhood sharing program.

4. With clothing, even if you really love something or wear it a lot, if it has holes or is wearing thin or has stains, see if you can part with it. Energetically, this is usually for the best. If you have sentimental attachment, if it's deeply cherished, consider taking a photo and/or writing about the memories associated with it, before tossing it out. Or you can repurpose some of it, such as by making a quilt or turning it into a dust rag. You may

also want to consider the material. Is it synthetic? Natural? Does it allow your skin pores to breathe?

5. Go through every part of your living space, work space, and car if applicable. Remember to take your time and break it down into manageable chunks of time and spaces. Just keep at it until you've gotten rid of as much excess as you can.

6. Although this might not feel necessary right after a big decluttering project, consider getting rid of one thing for each new thing you bring in to your home. This may not work in all situations, but it works well for things like books or clothing and can be a great maintenance plan after doing a big clearing.

7. If there are things you're not ready to part with yet, Laura Lavigne suggests boxing that stuff up, putting a date on the box, and giving it another year. Ideally store that box somewhere out of the house, like in a garage or storage shed. And if you haven't gone to it to take anything out, when that year is up, just give it all away.

8. If you live with others who aren't on board with decluttering? Have a conversation with them about the benefits and what it would mean to you. You could also frame it as an experiment—or even a game (for example, if children are involved). Be open to negotiating, and do what you can.

Follow these tips, and your home environment will transform. You'll feel a sense of spaciousness that is not just physical, but also energetic. You'll feel as if some weight has been lifted. You'll also use this as an opportunity to examine—and get rid of—products that are truly toxic or otherwise unhealthy, when you go through your fridge, your pantry, your cleaning products, and your body-care products.

Non-Toxic Cleaning and Body-Care Products

At last! It's time to revisit detoxing the body while decluttering, by assessing your body-care and cleaning products. There are many products commonly used on our bodies and to clean our homes that contain ingredients we're better off avoiding. Sure, our bodies are designed to handle a certain amount of toxins without getting sick. But why not use only the cleanest and purest products possible? This is not only best for our bodies, but also best for our planet.

I can already hear one possible answer, though: cost.

Yes, it's true that many of the "natural" or "green" products cost more, but not all of them. Plus, there are green cleaning and body-care hacks that cut costs, such as:

- **Baking soda:** Do you know how much you can do with baking soda?! You can clean your home with it. You can brush your teeth with it. You can even use it to wash your hair. The list goes on—and I've included a link to that list in the Resources section.
- **Vinegar:** Like baking soda, there's a lot you can do with vinegar that will actually save you money. For example, on its own or combined with baking soda, vinegar is also a wonderful natural cleaner. And apple cider vinegar can be used as a conditioning rinse in your hair!
- **Coconut oil:** Although some people say it clogs their pores, if it doesn't clog yours, this is what I recommend as a face and body moisturizer. It can also be used as a mouthwash by using it for oil pulling with some clove oil or other essential oil added to it. Be sure to consult with a doctor if using essential oils internally—even though you're not swallowing it, clove oil may be contraindicated in some cases, such as if you're pregnant.
- **Dr. Bronner's Pure Castile Liquid Soap:** This stuff can be used for a variety of home and body cleaning. You can use it as bodywash or shampoo, as laundry

detergent, as dishwashing liquid, to clean your floors
or your countertops, and more!

For tips on how to use these products, check out the Resources section.

One of the cool things about switching over to using these
products on their own, or combining them with other ingredients to create natural cleaning and body-care products, is that it
will also result in decluttering! Fewer products for multiple
purposes means less stuff! Less stuff to buy. Less stuff taking up
space. And less stuff for you to manage and be responsible for
means you will have more energy and feel lighter and brighter!

A Note About Sunscreen

Speaking of brightness, when I started using purer products on
my skin many years ago, I felt a bit stumped in the realm of
sunscreen. I was such a health nut about it back then that I
didn't want to put any moisturizer on my skin that I wouldn't
feel comfortable eating! So, what was I to do about sun
protection?

In recent years, there's been more information about what's
healthiest in terms of sunscreen, and I have let go of that edible
requirement. Plus, dermatologists don't recommend coconut oil
as sunscreen, and I'm pretty sure I got burned once because
of it!

Now I mostly look for sunscreens that have titanium
dioxide or zinc oxide as their active ingredient, because those
are considered the safest. I'm not always super strict in this
department, such as if I'm traveling and need to buy sunscreen
someplace where my options are limited. What you choose to
do about sunscreens—and other products—depends on you
and your level of chemical sensitivity or concern. Sometimes
you need to weigh the risks and benefits, and you might not

always choose, or have access to, the most "natural" product every time. But, when possible, I recommend you choose the purest, least toxic sunscreen available. I also recommend checking out the Environmental Working Group's sunscreen information. They're the ones who also put out that Dirty Dozen list each year. You can learn all about sunscreen ingredients from them at www.ewg.org/sunscreen.

For additional protection, you can also wear clothing that acts as sunscreen and a hat with a visor to shade your face. But don't rely on that alone. Check out that EWG site, and find a sunscreen you like that's approved by them.

Products and Ingredients to Avoid?

As you start decluttering your body-care and cleaning products, look at the ingredients. I say that if you can't pronounce it, then you probably don't want to use it. Even some things we *can* pronounce are harmful! When shopping for new products, and when cleaning out what you already have, here are some basic things to avoid and eliminate completely or at least reduce:

- Sulfates
- Phytates
- Phthalates
- Ammonia
- Chlorine
- Triclosan
- Perchloroethylene, or "PERC"
- Quaternary ammonium compounds, or "QUATS"
- 2-Butoxyethanol
- Sodium hydroxide

How extreme you want to be with this is up to you. When it comes to body-care and cleaning products, I tend to apply that

80/20 rule we looked at in the Body chapter. For example, although most of my cleaning products don't contain the ingredients listed above, a couple times a month I do use products like Tilex spray or Clorox wipes in my bathroom and kitchen, with windows open and fans on for good ventilation.

Since I am not totally strict about this in my own life, and since chemical toxins are not my area of expertise, I am not going to go into detail about this list. I just want to provide a little information, to plant a seed about something for you to consider. And if you'd like to learn more—if you feel this is an important aspect of detoxing *your* life—then I recommend you read the article "8 Hidden Toxins: What's Lurking in Your Cleaning Products."

In the Resources section, you can find a link to that article and other information on chemical toxins and how to detox your home—and not just in terms of body-care and cleaning products but even things like paint, mattresses, curtains, and rugs. Yes, if you are extra sensitive to chemicals or have some mysterious health ailment, you might want to dive deeper into this topic, starting with the recommended reading at the end of this book.

Pollution

Another aspect of home detoxing is the air you breathe. Swapping out toxic cleaning products for natural ones and eliminating chemical fragrances from your home environment will help. And surely you already know that "getting fresh air" is good for you. But how fresh is that air even if you're using all-natural products?

If there have been forest fires blowing smoke your way, if the pollution level is high in your city, or you live by a freeway, consider limiting the amount of time you keep your windows open—and find a good air purifier and regularly change the filters. Once again, I'm going to direct you to the good ol' Environmental Working Group, at www.ewg.org/healthyhomeguide. Diving deep into the topic of air filters goes beyond my expertise and the scope of this book, but EWG is a great place to start if you'd like to research this subject.

Before we move on, though, just a note about houseplants. Some say they are like mini natural air purifiers. Some say that's not really true. While I wouldn't recommend houseplants *in place of* a good air filtration system, I say why not see if it makes you feel better having more greenery around you! The science may not support that investing in houseplants can counteract pollution and enhance air quality, but plants do take in carbon dioxide and emit oxygen. Plus, they help us connect with nature, which can be both soothing and energizing. In articles that recommend houseplants for air purification, here are some of the top runners:

- Barberton daisy
- English ivy
- Snake plant
- Chrysanthemum
- Spider plant
- Aloe vera
- Broadleaf lady palm
- Dragon tree
- Weeping fig
- Chinese evergreen

Note: Some of these plants may be toxic to your pets. Consult with your vet. I also visit the APSCA website (link in resources) before bringing new plants into my home—or my backyard.

Why Bother?

Why bother doing any of this? Why switch products? Why declutter? Does it really matter? Does it really make a difference? Will it be worth it?

Detoxing and decluttering your home might feel like a big project—even if you feel excited about it and enjoy things like decluttering or learning how to use all-natural products. So get clear on what you're willing and wanting to take on, and then be sure to break it down into manageable tasks to avoid overwhelm or self-sabotage. I tend to want to do things like this quickly and all at once. And sometimes I have the time and energy to dedicate to that, so I can relate if you have that urge. But please set yourself up for success by being realistic about what you can do and when you can do it and how much change to implement at once.

Being clear on the benefits will inspire and motivate you. Then you just need to schedule it in and commit to following through. You can also pick and choose what advice you want to take. Maybe you don't want to switch to more natural body-care products, but do want to eliminate toxic cleaning products or just get rid of excess material possessions. Or maybe you want non-toxic products but actually prefer to keep your clutter! Some people feel more joy with more stuff around, and that's totally fine. You can still declutter the "hidden" spaces, like drawers and cabinets, to derive some decluttering benefits. Whatever feels best for you. You have total freedom of choice here. But either way, consider the following:

Benefits of decluttering:

- Less material stuff means less responsibility—and less dust! Letting go of excess responsibility lightens you up and frees up your energy so it can flow better.

- A greater sense of freedom! With your energy and time freed up, thanks to less clutter and less stuff, you will feel more of a general sense of freedom.
- More energy! The less stuff in your environment, and the better organized it is without clutter, the better energy flows around you. This helps your own energy flow. Plus, you'll have more energy with fewer things to manage, less input taking up space in that mental computer of yours.
- More joy! You will feel a greater sense of joy with this increase of energy and freedom, a feeling of burdens lifted thanks to getting rid of excess stuff.
- A sense of expansion! With more free and clear space around you, you'll tap into a sense of expansiveness, which helps you see more possibilities for yourself and feel open and receptive for what you truly want for yourself and your life.
- Greater self-awareness! As you go through the process of decluttering, you'll learn some things about yourself and what really matters to you. You'll also become more aware of how material things affect your thoughts and feelings and your overall sense of well-being.

When you declutter, you detox your environment. You free up your energy. You have more time and space. And it is one of the easiest ways to start detoxing your life. You might even choose to focus on home decluttering before you try to detox your body or your mind. As always, it is up to you!

Benefits of non-toxic products include:

- Healthier skin
- Better air quality, resulting in happier lungs
- More energy and an enhanced immune system, because your body isn't as busy trying to process toxins you inhale or absorb into your skin
- Feeling good about also being more environmentally friendly

There you have it! Some decluttering advice. Some product guidance. And some reminders of the benefits you're looking for—whether it's through detoxing your home, your body, your mind, or your relationships, when you detox your life, you'll feel better. Remember to focus on how you want to feel and what you want your life to be. It's important to remember that especially as we enter into the next chapter: Relationships!

RELATIONSHIPS

RELATIONSHIPS ARE a big part of life. Not just romantic relationships. All relationships. There is no question that close and ongoing relationships affect our overall sense of well-being. And even one-time, short-term, or otherwise limited interactions can affect us, for better or for worse—and sometimes both. Relationships can be a big source of joy and pleasure, but they can also be an energy drain or block us from feeling, doing, and being our best.

Now that you've learned a bit about how to clean and clear your body, your mind, and your material world, it's time to put some of that knowledge—and some additional tips—into practice in your interpersonal world. Because relationships are so important in our lives, it's crucial to clean up those that need to be cleaned, and possibly to let some go if that's truly what's best. In this chapter, we explore how to do this—how to detox our relationships.

But how do you know if a relationship is "toxic"?

For starters, do you feel drained when you are with this person, or after being with them? Do you feel anxious? Do you fight a lot? Do you feel disrespected, manipulated, neglected, used, or gaslit? Have you received the silent treatment? Do you walk on eggshells? Do you feel avoidant? If you answer yes to any of these questions, it's time for a detox—or at least a closer look.

Detoxing relationships doesn't always mean declaring someone else, or a relationship, *toxic*, and then just cutting people out of your life. Although it certainly can result in that, sometimes detoxing a relationship is more about making the relationship healthier, such as by setting healthy boundaries, clearing up misunderstandings, learning better communication skills, and being honest about what's really going on— including looking at your own role in the toxic dynamic. Unless it's a downright *abusive* relationship, ending a relationship completely is a last resort, after it's clear that no matter how much you try to detox it, it's just not a healthy dynamic.

As the saying goes, it takes two to tango. However, if you're being physically or verbally abused, no victim blaming here; your only job is to look at how to safely leave that dance, not how to dance differently so that the abuser stops. And even when there's not actual *abuse* occurring, it's perfectly fine to walk away, as sometimes that is the best and healthiest choice. It's even okay to burn some bridges as you walk away if that's what it takes to keep you healthy and safe.

Before we look at how to detox relationships, first let's clear something up to prevent creating even more toxicity while attempting to detox.

NOTE: If you're in an abusive relationship, you can use this book for supplemental support, but please get professional support from an organization like the National Domestic Violence Hotline: 1–800–799–7233 or TTY 1-800-787-3224, www.thehotline.org.

The Problem with Labeling People as Toxic

Over the past few years, I've questioned if, in the realm of relationships, the word "toxic" is overused and therefore could be creating even more toxicity. I've questioned if people can really be considered intrinsically "toxic," and I'm not so sure. It seems to me that personal or relational toxicity may depend more on the circumstances and that we are all capable of being perceived (or misperceived) as "toxic," being mislabeled (or accurately labeled) as narcissistic, and contributing to an unhealthy dynamic.

The person you view as "toxic" just might also be viewing you as toxic too. It's natural for the human brain to deflect blame and assign it to others. And it's natural to want to condemn someone for harmful behavior that hurt you. But *labeling* someone as toxic just might *be* toxic. Does it really do any good? Does it do more harm than good?

Maybe it actually does do good by helping you recognize how unhealthy the relationship is or how much you don't want that person in your life. But do your best not to demonize others or yourself when recognizing toxic patterns. You can, instead, recognize our shared humanity while also making healthy changes to improve your communication and boundaries.

Of course, in some cases, the way someone treats you may be something you absolutely know you would never do to someone else. And sometimes we have to go through an angry stage in which "demonizing the other" is part of our process. But the thing to remember here is that it's meant to be just one part of the process we move through on our way to a sense of peace and freedom that can be achieved through healthy boundaries and forgiveness—or at least some compassion and acceptance, even if disengaged and from afar.

We all have our struggles and flaws. It doesn't make poor

treatment okay, but it can take the edge off a bit to remember that—to remember our shared humanity.

Now, let's start looking at how to discern whether a relationship just needs to be cleansed or if it needs to be totally purged.

Is the Relationship Salvageable?

Although sometimes total disengagement and cutting ties is the best and healthiest choice, sometimes toxic relationships can be transformed into healthy relationships. In order to detox a relationship, you can start by improving how you interact with these people—as long as it truly is safe to stay in a relationship with them while seeing if things could change for the better.

In some circumstances, you can make clear requests to others about their behavior. Sometimes having a heart-to-heart about what you're experiencing is what's needed, if it feels physically and emotionally safe to do so. The tricky thing here is that after experiencing certain types of harm in a relationship, the vulnerability of having a heart-to-heart may not feel right. Consulting with a therapist, a mediator, or some other trusted and objective third party could be helpful in determining what would be best.

And in cases of extreme toxicity (for example, when narcissism or borderline personality disorder are in the mix), unfortunately, these conversations usually don't lead to change, or at least not sustainable change. Sometimes talking even backfires and results in things like gaslighting and manipulation—or worse, such as escalation to a verbal or physical attack. Again, some sort of third-party involvement is recommended in cases like this, both for supportive guidance and for safety.

In my own life, sometimes it has taken objective third parties to help me recognize when I've been gaslit or emotionally manipulated in other ways—and to recognize things like narcissism, whether full blown or just somewhere on the spectrum (more on narcissism below). I had to learn the hard way that not everyone deserves to hear my heart; sometimes it's best to just disengage. And to forgive from afar. Not every toxic relationship dynamic can be transformed simply by calling it out—or calling it *in* to integrity. And not every relationship you may choose to disengage from is *toxic;* sometimes things just shift, and people grow apart. This chapter focuses more on toxic relationships than on relationships that just change or fizzle out. It's also not just about romantic relationships. Friendships, professional relationships, and family are all part of this. As you continue reading, and if you use the assessment practice that's coming up, my hope is that you will get better at discerning which relationships can be cleaned up and transformed for the better—and which cannot.

Finding the Gifts, and Letting Go with Love

There can be some tough calls to make here. And sometimes it takes time and experimenting to determine what is best when trying to clean up—or completely clear out—a toxic relationship.

Although I used to be someone who always wanted to talk things out, even if at first I felt avoidant, I've learned that with *some* people it's best to just walk away, to not talk it out, to not share my heart or make requests. It has felt uncomfortable at times to do things in this different way, to *not* try to work stuff out, to not try to fix what's broken or stay friends with certain people. But deep down I do know it's been for the best, and I've learned and grown so much by facing these relational challenges and choosing to handle them in ways that go beyond my comfort zone.

I now see that sometimes walking away from people, even if they weren't downright abusive, is a form of self-care and self-love. And that makes me better able to support others, like you, in making the tough choice of disengagement. Or perhaps your comfort zone is disengagement, and your growth edge will be learning to talk stuff out.

Either way, finding the gifts in these difficult situations is also a loving form of self-care and part of personal growth. Finding the gratitude and the lessons that come from having moved through a toxic relationship can soothe and balance out the challenging aspects. You might want to journal about this and make a list of gifts, growth, and lessons learned when contemplating your past and current relationships.

You can also consider how the other person may be a gift in other people's lives. It might feel uncomfortable to do so at first, or if the wounds are too fresh, but sometimes it's helpful depending on the circumstances and where you're at in your process. Some of the most toxic relationships I've experienced have been with people who have been great influences on other people's lives as friends, lovers, therapists, and even as "healers." Oftentimes, I started out thinking they were a gift in *my* life. Then I'd feel like they were the opposite of a gift! But eventually I could find the gifts again.

After some time of going through the grief process, of letting go of the toxicity, there was some softening and gratitude around the positive aspects of what I experienced before things got ugly. And you can have this experience of softening and recognition too. It may take some time, but it's possible. And healing.

So if you need to cut someone out of your life, just try your best to do it with love and compassion—even if you don't like the person. We all have our shit. Let go with love—even if it's just love for yourself. Let walking away be an act of self-love and self-care, filling yourself up with so much love for yourself that there is not even room to hate or resent the other person.

As the saying goes, "hurt people hurt people." It's not

personal. And you don't need to give that person access to your life. You can disengage. You can take your power back. You can love, without liking, and be compassionate from afar.

One way of creating some spaciousness and softening into compassion is through Sheng Zhen, those meditation and qigong practices for opening the heart and cultivating not only qi but also unconditional love. Although all Sheng Zhen practices help with this, a movement called Unraveling the Heart comes to mind here as a simple and easy one to share with you for cultivating compassion and holding space for all you're feeling as you detox your relationships.

I've created an Unraveling the Heart bonus video for you, so if you'd like to pause reading here to go check that out, please do at www.rebeccacliogould.com/detoxbonuses. Otherwise, let's continue on with assessing your relationships to get you more clear on what needs some cleaning up and/or which relationships might need to end. And then we'll discuss how to improve your remaining relationships through things like energy clearing, communication, and boundaries.

Assessing the Situation

Before deciding what kind of communication and boundaries are needed, and whether the relationship can be detoxed and transformed or just needs to end, it's important to assess the situation. It's crucial to identify what's yours and what's theirs. Sometimes we stay in toxic dynamics because we're taking on too much responsibility or blame. Conversely, sometimes we don't recognize our own part and instead project it all onto the other.

While we don't want to assign excessive or unfair blame to others, and we do want to take personal responsibility for our own role in things, we also don't want to take on *too much* responsibility. Just be real about your part in a toxic dynamic, without taking on more than what is yours. Honesty is always the best policy, so if you have any toxic relationships in your life, or suspect some toxicity, it's time to take an honest look at what's really going on. And then you can figure out the best detox method for your particular situation.

ACTIVITY:
WHOSE SHIT IS THIS? AND HOW BAD IS IT?

Set aside some time, think of a troubling relationship, and ask yourself the following questions. Write down your answers. Write as much or as little as you like, but do write instead of just thinking about it. You also have the option of coming back to this at the end of the chapter, or going through it now *and* later. It could be interesting to see if your answers evolve or become clearer after reading more.

- What habits, beliefs, or behaviors of the other person are contributing to the toxicity or harm to me and/or others?
- What habits, beliefs, or behaviors of mine are contributing to the toxicity or harm to myself and/or others? *Please note: when looking at your own possible toxicity, try not to shame and blame yourself. This is just about taking an honest look at how you might be contributing to the toxic dynamic.*
- Can it change for the better? If yes or maybe, how, and whose responsibility is it?
- Do I need to distance myself just a bit, or do I need to completely cut ties? Or something in between?
- Do we need a mediator to be part of a conversation to try to work this out, can we do it on our own, or is there no point in having the conversation (in

other words, is it unsafe physically or emotionally)?

- Now that I've answered these questions, what's my next best step?

If you need time to sit with your answers before knowing your next step, or before acting on it, that is totally fine. If you're crystal clear and ready for your next step right away, go for it. And if you've determined you need a mediator or some other third party to help with this? Find one. You can also go through this process again, to further refine your answers, after reading the remainder of this chapter.

How to Handle Difficult People, Including Yourself!

Now that you've started to look at what's yours and what's not yours, what's next? How to handle difficult people so that you don't feel so entangled, reactive, or drained? And how to handle yourself, if you've recognized that sometimes you're the difficult person?

What you've learned in the Mind chapter can be really helpful when it comes to dealing better with others—and with yourself. There are also a variety of tools we'll explore in this chapter, such as clear communication and boundary setting, "energy hygiene," and mindful breathing.

If you already have a meditation practice, or have decided to implement one thanks to my earlier suggestion to do so, fantastic! I also recommend taking a few minutes at the start of each day with some energy cleaning and clearing to increase and enhance the quality of your energy. In times of distress, things like meditation and energy hygiene practices bring you back to yourself and your body instead of being all up in your head, thinking about the difficult person or situation. You may want to create an energy bubble or protective shield to help you stay more centered and clean and clear in your own energy. And you can try it now with the following practice.

ACTIVITY:
ENERGY EGG

In 2018 energy-healer Elke Siller Macartney taught me her Energy Egg practice. And I've been using it ever since. This is how I do it:

1. Stand comfortably, with soft knees and straight back.
2. Imagine there are two pillars coming up from the ground for the palms of your hands to rest on.
3. Imagine an energy egg (an egg-shaped energy field) around you. You can picture the energy like light or some other visual. See that its edges are about three feet away from your body. And feel or imagine this energy egg really grounding into the earth so that the part beneath your feet is a few feet below you.
4. Clean and clear your energy egg. You can do so simply by thinking "clean and clear" several times. Alternatively or additionally, you can intentionally move your hands through the space as if clearing cobwebs or incorporate a short qigong practice called Gathering Qi. *See video in the bonus material.*
5. If you want some added protection, such as prior to engaging with someone "toxic" or being around people who are sick, you can add on the "Shields Up" practice: create a semi-permeable energy shield around you simply by imagining it. Visualize it. Feel it. Believe it's there. And know that only what's good, only what you allow, can come in.

I've been using this practice since the day Elke taught it to me, and I love it. I usually also spray some rosewater over myself before, during, or after. It makes me feel centered and grounded, embodied, and clear. It can also help you feel like you have *more* energy. When you have a clean and clear energy egg around you, you're less likely to get energy drained or energy zapped, which means you'll feel more vibrant and joyful, and more at peace.

The energy egg practice can protect you from other people's energy, but what about when you're energetically entangled with someone?

One of the things that can make detoxing relationships so tricky is energetic cords. *What are energetic cords?* They are strands of energy that connect us to others and are formed through our interactions. And even if you don't believe in things like energy strands, simply imagining them can be helpful in cleaning up connections with others. Think of it like this: There are positive cords, and there are negative cords. Usually, when there's toxicity, people want to cut the cords.

However, sometimes cutting cords isn't really what's best. It could be that more of a gentle dissolve is called for. Or perhaps just detangling the cords. I've cut or dissolved cords before, and then sometimes wondered if simply detangling them would have been better.

Jen Eramith, a spiritual teacher, was the one who taught me about detangling rather than cutting or dissolving. This is helpful in relationships that are "special" and can actually have healthy cording as long as you're disentangled.

ACTIVITY:
DETANGLING CORDS

Picture the cords like hairs flowing between your body

and the other person's body. Whenever you think of this
person, rather than trying to stop yourself from thinking
about them or trying to cut the cords, instead imagine
brushing or combing through the cords to detangle
them.

When I took Jen's advice and tried this detangling practice, it
worked. I stopped obsessing or feeling triggered. I didn't feel
the need to communicate with this other person, but I also
didn't feel the need to avoid. I didn't need to cut the ties. I just
needed the energy to be freed up to flow more smoothly, which
eventually allowed them to gently dissolve on their own.

But I do believe cutting or intentional dissolving is necessary in some situations. For cutting, you can imagine scissors
cutting the cords. And then call back your energy into yourself
and visualize filling with light afterwards. For gentle dissolving,
I highly recommend Lisa Beachy's Energy Cord Cutting Meditation on YouTube (see Resources section). If it doesn't resonate
with you, try some others. You can also hire an energy healer,
such as Elke Macartney, to clean your energy field.

Using these energy practices truly can help you better
handle challenging people and situations. Even if you're not so
sure about all this "energy" stuff, just give it try. Use your imagi-
nation to picture the energy like light, and just open up to the
possibility that it's real and can help you.

Mindful breathing is also supportive here. When thinking
about the relationship or feeling triggered in another person's
presence, take a deep breath and remember that it's not your
job to fix or satisfy the difficult person. Stay out of their busi-
ness as much as possible by *not* trying to control, micromanage,
or change them. Recognize what is not your responsibility as
well as what is. Bring one hand or both hands to your heart,
take a breath, and take a moment to feel some compassion for
that person and for yourself. Be kind without being a doormat

—be sure to do what you need to do to stand up for yourself and protect yourself from harm. Oftentimes, disengaging is key.

When possible, avoid silent treatment, though. Silent treatment is a toxic behavior that should only be used if somebody is being abusive and not respecting your clearly stated boundaries around communication. You can disengage without going completely silent—or if total silence feels necessary, then first let the other person know or ask a third party to clearly communicate that there will be no contact. What we really want here is a "less is more" approach when faced with triggering or draining behavior or communication from another person. Do your best to de-escalate the situation, which usually means minimal or zero engagement. Don't let them hook you. Don't try to hook them. And when possible, only communicate when not feeling triggered or agitated.

It's also okay to tell people you need some time and space. It's healthy to clearly communicate something like that. Do what you need to do for yourself in order to have a healthier dynamic—even if just while sorting out how to totally end this relationship in a way that doesn't do more harm.

And when you feel full of negativity, whether it's because of your own thoughts and energy, or because somebody else's toxicity oozed over into your personal bubble? Clearing your energy field can be helpful. If you're feeling too negative to think clearly about what the healthiest course of action would be, you can use the Energy Egg practice above or try the Sheng Zhen practices or guided meditation in the bonus material.

I've already mentioned Unraveling the Heart, and that's a great one for holding space for your own emotions, as well as for allowing your heart to clean and clear your energy and emotions. Another one of my favorite Sheng Zhen movements for transforming or removing negativity is called Expelling Unhealthy Qi. (See the bonus materials for a video.) The movement itself is useful, and the contemplation can help you main-

tain or embrace a more positive attitude while in the process of
expelling unhealthy qi—and therefore it can also apply to
removing unhealthy relationships from your life:

*There must be a sense of relaxation in letting the unhealthy qi go.
One must not look upon the unhealthy qi with loathing or as something dirty, but rather as that which when released will leave space
in the body for fresh qi. The unhealthy qi is only unhealthy
depending on the circumstances in which it is found. But as soon as it
is released, it becomes neutral once again.* —from A Return to
Oneness

Isn't that a beautiful message? Through practicing this
movement and contemplating these words, you'll begin to relax
into the letting go. And harsh or negative feelings will melt
away into a place of neutrality—or perhaps even love. You'll be
better able to handle "difficult" people—including yourself!

Compassionate Detachment

One way in which toxicity gets created is through attachments.
By learning to detach, with compassion, we can have healthier
relationships. And if the relationship still needs to end, then
compassionate detachment helps us end the relationship more
gracefully and with less pain.

Be careful not to create more toxicity by thinking nasty
thoughts about someone you had a toxic relationship with. But
don't beat yourself up over those thoughts if they do arise;
sometimes that's part of the process. And it's a great opportunity for compassionate detachment.

How to compassionately detach? When you think of the
other person or a troubling situation, or when those negative
thoughts arise or you feel triggered, be compassionate with
yourself and gently let it be to then let it go. The Unraveling the

Heart practice is supportive for this too. There's also the following practice I learned from Kathianne Lewis at the Center for Spiritual Living in Seattle. I highly recommend this practice and can vouch for its effectiveness.

ACTIVITY:

I LOVE YOU, I BLESS YOU, I RELEASE YOU

This isn't something you communicate directly to the other person. This is something you say silently (or out loud, if alone) to get clean and clear with yourself. Here's what you do:

Hold the person in your mind and repeat the words, "I love you. I bless you. I release you." Or, "I love you. I bless you. I let you live your own life." And for maximum effectiveness, for really sticky situations, try the 70 x 7 approach. Repeat this seventy times, for seven days, with the person in mind. Another way to amp it up is to include a body movement or gesture for each part. *For a video demonstration, see book bonuses.*

Alternative wording: Although the way Kathianne Lewis taught it worked well for me, I have also thought about other options. If you really can't get behind the words above, you can just say, "I forgive you." Or "I forgive myself." Or "Thank you." Or "Thank you for what you've taught me. We are done now. Goodbye." To prepare for this alternative version, you might first need to think about what you've learned from this challenging experience so that you feel good—and authentic—about what you're saying.

You might need to "fake it until you make it" with this practice. But if you give it a chance, it truly can shift things for the better. It can free you from feeling weighed down and burdened by whatever happened in the relationship.

Protecting Yourself Without Being Overprotective

Once we become more aware of toxic relationships, sometimes we become overprotective or hypervigilant. Although sometimes walls need to go up or bridges need to be burned, other times we just need healthier boundaries in place! By implementing the following suggestions, you just might see a toxic relationship *detox* and transform into a healthy relationship.

Here's what I suggest:

- Take some time to clarify your needs and boundaries and values. Get out a journal or notebook and make some lists.
- Cultivate an open heart, and practice being more embodied. Use breath to come back into your body when you notice tape loop or negative thoughts. And practice heart-opening meditation practices, such as Sheng Zhen.
- When someone makes a request of you or extends an invitation, it's okay to say you'll get back to them the next day—or within twenty-four hours (or two or three days, depending on the context). You can also ask the other person to check back with you if you haven't gotten back to them by a specified date.
- Take more time for yourself to reflect and recharge.
- Practice clearer communication about your feelings and needs.
- Get comfortable saying no. No is a full sentence in and of itself. But if "no" is hard for you, keep reading...

Just Say No

Each item listed above could have its own section, or even its own chapter! But that's not the kind of book this is. And yet I feel we need to spend some more time on saying no, because I know it can be hard—and because it's such an essential part of having healthier boundaries as you detox your life. Saying no is crucial in relationships, and it also applies to the material we covered in the previous chapters.

First of all, I want you to recognize that you deserve to have boundaries, and your boundaries are beautiful. They're important. If someone doesn't like or can't respect your boundaries, that is their problem. It doesn't mean you shouldn't have those boundaries. But you do need to do your part by clarifying and communicating your boundaries. We can't always just expect others to know what our boundaries are if we don't tell them. And, unfortunately, sometimes we don't know what boundaries we need in place until they've been violated.

Even when someone has violated a boundary, although you have a right to be angry, consider if this was part of you learning about how to have clearer and better boundaries. Of course there are some boundaries that seem as if they'd be obvious—like expecting that a stranger isn't going to grope you. Some boundaries may be a given; others need to be communicated. Sometimes that communication is direct: for example, "Please don't text me multiple times before I've had a chance to reply to the first text." Other times the communication is indirect: for example, sharing your email address, but not your phone number, with potential clients.

Another type of boundary violation that can arise, and that we may not be aware of until it happens, is when people ask questions that feel too personal. That can feel so icky, even if their intentions are good. It's okay to not answer, as doing so would mean violating your own boundaries. Try saying something like, "I'd rather not answer that," or "That feels too personal to share (right now)." Don't feel obligated. The icky feeling may even have less to do with that other person and have more to do with your potential to violate your own boundaries if you're not feeling grounded and clear in them.

One of the worst boundary violations is when we violate ourselves by choosing to say or do something that doesn't really feel right, just because someone else is asking for it. It's okay to say no, and you don't even have to explain. But it can be helpful for some types of people to be told when a question they've asked is too personal; it can help them learn, or at least help them understand your reaction. Communicating about these types of things can keep your relationship clean and clear by not withholding your feeling of discomfort and the reason why you don't want to answer or don't want to do whatever you're being asked to do. But it's totally up to you how much or how little you say.

And one of the most important skills in communicating your boundaries and respecting your own boundaries? Getting comfortable with saying *no*!

No can help you detox a relationship. *No* can help you disengage. *No* can help you relate in a healthier way. *No* can help you walk away.

It's okay to say *no*. It's essential to be able to say *no*. Saying *no* is also saying *yes*, saying yes to what's truly best for you by saying no to what is not.

If saying no is hard for you, you can start building your skills by first buying yourself some time. Sometimes the hard part is even recognizing that we *want* to say no, if we respond too quickly with a yes. To buy yourself some time to either get clear on what you really want or to prepare yourself to say no, all you have to do is say one of the following:

- *I'll need to get back to you tomorrow on that.*

- *Let me get back to you in a day or two.*
- *I'm not sure, but I can let you know tomorrow (or by the end of today).*

I also love Marcia Baczynski's list of twelve ways to say no. Although no is a complete sentence, and you certainly don't need to use any of these suggestions, in some situations these might feel supportive and like great ways to say no in a way that helps both you and the other person still feel a good connection—not that you're obligated to do that. It's just an option, depending on who you're interacting with and what you're being asked, and what you want or don't want moving forward. Here's Marcia's list, and in the Resources section, you can find a link to her article on saying no gracefully:

- I'm a no to that, but I'm a yes to you.
- I'm not so into that, but you go have fun!
- I want to be in connection with you, but that doesn't work for me. Can we do this instead?
- I'm a no for now.
- Not tonight.
- I'm not available for anything like that right now.
- I need to build more trust before I'd be willing to consider that.
- No, thank you.
- Not today.
- I don't have the internal resources to pull that off.
- IImmmm... That's not going to work.
- It's really hard for me to say no to people, but I'm practicing being braver and more honest, so I'm going to say no right now.

For relationships that can be transformed rather than

ended, learning how to say no and feeling comfortable and even loving as you say it, can be a total game changer.

ACTIVITY:
GETTING TO NO AND KNOWING YOUR BOUNDARIES

Clear communication about your boundaries and expectations detoxes relationships and prevents energy drains.

Step 1: Get clear on what boundaries you want and need. How to do this? Think about what feels good to you and/or what hasn't felt good. When did you feel your boundaries were violated or you wished you'd had clearer or stronger boundaries in place?

Step 2: Practice how you want to communicate these boundaries to others, if they are boundaries to be communicated out loud or in writing. Write down how you would say it to get clearer and feel more comfortable stating your boundaries. If you feel uncomfortable, ask a good friend or a therapist to be on the receiving end of hearing your boundaries, and ask them to validate your boundaries by agreeing to them and appreciating or thanking you for your clarity and for communicating your needs.

Step 3: If boundaries have been violated, it might be necessary to request a conversation in which you address that and now clarify your boundaries. Otherwise, many boundaries come up more situationally and need to be expressed on an as-needed basis.

Optional: Practice saying no, out loud, in various ways. *Refer to Marcia Baczynski's list.*

Getting more comfortable saying no and setting boundaries will prevent energy drains and resentments, which create major toxicity when left to fester. As you clarify your boundaries and use your "no" more often, you'll find you have healthier, happier relationships, and more time and energy to enjoy them —and all of life!

A Note About Narcissism

If you find that despite your best efforts, things are just not getting better and maybe even getting worse, you may be dealing with a narcissist. Or with narcissistic behavior. Narcissism is a huge topic that goes *way* beyond the scope of my professional expertise—and this book. But it is worth mentioning briefly, because many toxic relationships involve full-blown narcissistic personality disorder or at least some narcissistic tendencies.

According to *The Diagnostic and Statistical Manual of Mental Disorders*, narcissistic personality disorder comprises a pervasive pattern of grandiosity (in fantasy or behavior), a constant need for admiration, and a lack of empathy. But please keep in mind that as a layperson, you really can't diagnose someone as a narcissist. The word "narcissist" certainly can be overused and misused when it comes to relationships. And some say that we all have some narcissism in us. There's a spectrum. Narcissistic characteristics can be displayed without there being an actual personality disorder.

Some people have full-blown personality disorders, but even they are not coming across as toxic *everywhere* they go and with *everyone* they meet. And occasionally someone else's narcissistic or harmful behavior may bring out narcissistic or other emotionally abusive or unhealthy behavior in you. It may even result in you asking yourself, *What if I'm the narcissist?* This question can be a result of the actual narcissist gaslighting you. But it can also be a reminder to look honestly at your own reactions and behavior.

Self-awareness and self-inquiry are essential when working on creating healthier relationships and cleaning up toxic relationship dynamics. Once you're clean and clear on your end, you'll be better able to see if the relationship can be healthy and continue, or if it's time to walk away. And if you are involved with a narcissist, or suspect you are, then you might want to get *un*involved—or get some professional help to support you.

Keeping the Heart Open

If through this process you discover you need to distance yourself from someone or completely cut ties, be sure to keep that precious heart of yours open. One of the main culprits of toxic relationship patterns? A closed, or overprotected, guarded heart. It creates stagnant qi and negative emotions. In order to have healthier relationships, you'll want to consider regularly cleaning and clearing your energy *and* balancing your emotions through heart-opening practices such as Sheng Zhen.

Opening the heart—and keeping it open—will help you gain more clarity, cultivate better discernment, experience more compassion, assist with forgiveness, and bring more joy to your life. Whether you want to clean up a toxic relationship or attract healthier relationships, keeping the heart open will improve your relationships. When we've experienced some toxicity in a relationship, it can be easy to shut down, to close the heart, to feel all kinds of discomfort and knots—or shut down and feel numb so you don't feel anything at all. Sheng Zhen can be one of your tools for detoxing current relationships and attracting healthier ones.

If you have identified any relationships that need a good cleansing or a full-on purge, don't rush it. Be gentle with yourself. Be patient. Be loving. Remember how much happier you'll be and how much more energy you'll have once you've detoxed your relationships. Remember the end goal. Know that you deserve it.

And check out the book bonuses for some heart-healing and heart-opening guided meditations and Sheng Zhen practice videos to support you along the way as you detox your relationships and detox your life.

PUTTING IT ALL TOGETHER

CONGRATULATIONS! You've made it through the main chapters. Maybe you've already started implementing some detox suggestions along the way, or perhaps you decided to read the whole book first with the intention of integrating it into your life after taking it all in.

Either way, I want this to be easy for you. I want this to feel good to you. And since we are all different in terms of what the best approach may be, I want to share some practical ways to start detoxing your life over the course of ten days. Please note that ten days is just a start. If any of this feels overwhelming or like too much too soon, slow it down. Extend it. Turn the ten days into twenty days, or thirty days. Set yourself up for success by giving yourself the time and space to make sustainable changes that stretch you but don't tear you.

Especially when it comes to decluttering, depending on how much stuff you have, this most likely will need to get stretched out over a longer period of time. And perhaps you'll phase out certain products and foods over time, rather than just giving them away or throwing them away all at once. You have options here. You could spend a whole month just working on physical decluttering before you do anything else. Or you could do a thirty-day social media detox, without committing to making any dietary or other changes during that time. And then after that social media detox, dive in to another part of your life that could use some detoxing

It's up to you. Trust yourself to know what's best for you—but remember to consult with a doctor when it comes to some of the body stuff.

As for the mind and relationship detoxing? Well, those are things that tend to be ongoing and can take quite a bit of time as well. But you can get started here and now, if you're ready. You can follow every suggestion listed for each day, or pick and choose. Start where it's easy. Do what feels good. Take it step by step.

Remember, the following sample plan is just one example of how this could look. Reading through it all at once might feel overwhelming, but it is just an overview to get you thinking about what's possible. This one brings in aspects from the Body, Mind, Home, and Relationships chapters. Depending on your goals, this plan may not be the perfect fit for getting started. You can find additional examples in the bonus material, including an editable one so you can create your own plan.

Ten-Day Sample Plan

Day 1

- Start drinking more water.
- Remove the foods that you don't want to eat. If you have a family, it's best to get them on board. Otherwise, put all foods you wish to avoid in another part of the pantry, fridge, and freezer—more out of sight for you.

Day 2

- Continue drinking more water.
- Start eating more veggies, especially greens.

Day 3

- Continue with more water and more veggies.
- Start decluttering your physical environment. Choose a manageable space that you can complete with the time you have. Use Laura Lavigne's "actively used or deeply cherished" mantra.

Day 4

- Continue with water, veggies, and decluttering. If decluttering only works for you on certain days, such as on the weekend, adjust this plan as needed. Or adjust your expectation for how much you accomplish in a decluttering session. Remember that even just going through one drawer is something. Little by little, it all adds up—or in this case, subtracts down as you continue getting rid of things!
- Start oil pulling, even just five to ten minutes if twenty is too much for you for now.

Day 5

- Continue with what you've been doing the past few days.
- Start noticing your thoughts. It's time to start detoxing your mind! When you notice a negative, harmful, self-limiting, or sabotaging thought, write

it down, and then write a new statement that is more positive.

Day 6

- Add lemon water into your morning routine, continuing to drink lots of water throughout the day, and eat more veggies while avoiding sugar, white flour, etc. Instead of lemon, you can use apple cider vinegar in your water.
- Continue noting any negative ways of thinking, coming up with more positive ones, and practicing the positive ones.

Day 7

- If you haven't already, start replacing cleaning and body-care products that have toxic ingredients. If you want to finish up some products, so as not to be wasteful, or to ease the financial burden of replacing everything at once, just upgrade when you're ready. Unless your health is compromised, such as by issues with your liver, kidney, intestines, urinary system, immune system, or lymphatic system, then your body can process daily toxins just fine while you slowly but surely make some changes to reduce daily toxin exposure.

Day 8

- Pay attention to how your relationships feel. If you already know there's some toxicity, start planning how to handle it. Do you need to end the relationship? Have a conversation? Detangle or cut cords? Start with some compassionate detachment, so that you can decide most clearly, from the heart, with the best intentions.

Day 9

- Start a meditation practice if you don't already have one. Use this time to totally clear your mind or to focus only on positive thoughts, affirmations, and visualizing what you want and how you want to feel.

Day 10

- It's time for a social media detox—and/or reduction of email checking and news-watching. Decide whether it will be extreme, cold-turkey style, or just a designated number of times or number of minutes. Commit to at least a week, but ideally thirty days.

There it is. One example of how to get started over the course of ten days. Depending on where you're at and what your goals are, detoxing your life may be more of a gradual and ongoing process. Or maybe you want to dive in with a more intensive approach, doing more of a physical detox and a big decluttering project right off the bat! Either way, just keep in mind that the mental detoxing and relationship detoxing is meant to be more gradual and ongoing, even though parts of it can be done right away, such as a social media detox.

There's no right or wrong way to do this. However, if you have a physical illness that would benefit from more extreme and more comprehensive detoxing, please do check out the

Resources section. If you're just wanting to feel a bit brighter and lighter, healthier, and more in the flow with more energy, then you'll see great results simply by implementing the suggestions in this book without any further reading.

Finally, one more reminder to be gentle with yourself. Even if taking a more extreme approach, always check in with yourself along the way. Big changes can create stress, and that's toxic itself. So give yourself plenty of time and space to adjust. You may even feel worse at first, especially if making big dietary modifications. But even the mind and relationship detoxing can take a toll because it can stir up some deep and dark stuff; plus, it can feel painful to let go of people and things or thoughts—even when they are harming us.

And remember that when detoxing your life feels tough and you question if it's worth it or you want to give up, keep your eye on the prize. List out your goals and benefits. Write up a commitment statement. Make the changes that will get you the results you want, but give yourself some flexibility, time, and space. And keep in mind that I am here for you if you want additional support.

You can find me at www.rebeccacliogould.com.

Happy detoxing!

RESOURCES

Please note:
The entire contents of this section can also online, with clickable links, at www.rebeccacliogould.com/detoxresources.

Book Bonuses:
To access your book bonuses, including guided meditations, energy hygiene and cultivation practices, worksheets, a Detox Your Life song list, and sample plans, visit www.rebeccacliogould.com/detoxbonuses.

Blog:
For up-to-date new resources and blog posts about things that didn't make it into this book, visit www.detoxyourlife.info

Cleanses

There are various cleanses that follow a strict protocol and that might be suitable depending on your health and goals. The following cleanses are ones I have explored personally. However, with the colon cleanse and the liver and gallbladder cleansing books, I did not follow *all* recommendations. At the time, I had just become a health coach and was experimenting on myself by picking and choosing which advice to follow. I'm sharing them here, though, because I remember thinking they were good books with great advice. **Please consult with a doctor before starting any of these cleanses.**

- Purium's 10 Day Cleanse: Purium recently changed their 10 Day Transformation into a 30-Day Transformation. However, the 10-Day option is still available, and it the one I've used multiple times. I'll be totally honest and say that I've had the restrictiveness backfire for me once or twice, but overall it's been a good experience. Purium products are pricey, but I do believe in their quality and effectiveness enough to recommend them. If you decide to try it out, you can use the clickable links I've provided on my website or visit www.ishoppurium.com and enter "elementalharmony" as a code to receive a discount.

- If you either know or suspect that parasites or candida are wreaking havoc with your physical health, there are various supplements that can help. However, without making dietary changes, the supplements won't be sufficient. I recommend Paul Pitchford's parasite purge or candida cleanse suggestions, which can be found in his book *Healing with Whole Foods: Asian Traditions and Modern Nutrition*. You can also explore these protocols with a coach like me who studied with Paul Pitchford.

- *Complete Colon Cleanse: The At-Home Detox Program to Restore Good Health, Boost Vitality, and Ensure Longevity* by Dr. Edward F. Group III

- *The Liver and Gallbladder Miracle Cleanse: An All-*

Natural, At-Home Flush to Purify and Rejuvenate Your Body by Andreas Moritz

You may also want to explore books by Anthony William, such as *Medical Medium Liver Rescue* and *Medical Medium Celery Juice.* I can vouch for the benefits of celery juice!

Note: Depending on your current state of health and type of cleanse you want to do, you might need to prepare for an intensive detox by gradually changing your diet with good nutrition so that your organs are functioning well enough to support your liver. Otherwise, the detox can backfire and result in toxins pouring into your blood and getting reabsorbed. Working with a doctor, a health coach like me, or with a Nutritional Therapy Practitioner such as my colleague Pamela Grant is advised.

Other Books You Might Like

The following were either referenced in this book or are additional books that could be beneficial if you'd like to dive deeper into subjects such as your subconscious mind, conscious communication, emotional eating, and food and mood.

- *The Power of Your Subconscious Mind* by Joseph Murray
- *Breaking the Habit of Being Yourself: How to Lose Your Mind and Create a New One* by Dr. Joe Dispenza
- *The Four Agreements: A Practical Guide to Personal Freedom (A Toltec Wisdom Book)* by Don Miguel Ruiz
- *Crucial Conversations: Tools for Talking When Stakes are High* by Kerry Patterson, Joseph Grenny, Ron MicMillan, and Al Switzler
- *The Multi-Orgasmic Diet: Embrace Your Sexual Energy*

and Awaken Your Senses for a Healthier, Happier, Sexier You by Rebecca Clio Gould
- *Food & Mood: The Complete Guide to Eating Well and Feeling Your Best* by Elizabeth Somer

Qigong and Meditation Resources

- My Classes: www.rebeccacliogould.com
- Sheng Zhen: www.shengzhen.org
- SRF Guided Meditations: https://yogananda.org/guided-meditations

Energy Hygiene and Healing

- Elke Macartney: www.elkespage.com
- Susan DuMett: www.auroramindandenergy.com
- Donna Eden's Daily Energy Routine video on YouTube
- Lisa Beachy's Archangel Michael - Energy Cord Cutting Meditation Video on YouTube

Additional Resources

As referenced in the Body and Home chapters, www.ewg.org is a wonderful resource for nontoxic living. Please also visit www.rebeccacliogould.com/detoxresources for links to articles, videos, products, and more info on the following:

- Why Organic?
- Dirty Dozen and Clean Fifteen
- How to flavor your water (Pamela Grant's nutrition blog)

- Oil pulling
- Dry skin brushing
- Sunscreen
- Hormone-disrupting chemicals to avoid
- Dr. Bronner's uses
- Cleaning product toxins
- Environmental Working Group's Healthy Home Guide
- Skin care ingredients to avoid
- Baking soda hacks
- Vinegar cleaning hacks
- Houseplants
- Plant toxicity for pets
- Laura Lavigne's Happiness School: This contains the Lighten Up material referenced in the Home chapter.
- Laura Lavigne's Magic of Essence: This teaches you how focusing more on how you want to feel can work all sorts of magic in your life, and therefore it assists with detoxing your life.
- Marcia Baczynski's article on saying no gracefully – includes pdf postcard graphic.
- Lasting Love Connection for articles, online programs, and relationship coaching.
- Domestic Violence Support and Healthy Relationships Education

*Remember to check out www.detoxyourlife.info
and visit www.rebeccacliogould.com/detoxresources for clickable
links and up-to-date resources.*

ACKNOWLEDGMENTS

Thanks to Kristen Tate, at the Blue Garret, for editing and formatting my book. You were my proofreader and behind-the-scenes publishing angel a few years ago, with my first book, and it was a pleasure to work with you again as my editor and book designer this time around!

Speaking of designer, thanks to my book cover designer, Constance Mears, for so many beautiful designs—and for speaking the language of "Essence vs Form" with me. It was a tough choice when we got down to the final few designs, because I really couldn't go wrong with any of them. I appreciated seeing what it would look like to have a cover that matched my first book as well as covers that really spoke to this book's essences: simple, clean, easy, light, and bright!

Thanks to those who read my manuscript before the final editing phase: Daniel Gould, Pamela Grant, Dr. Jane Tornatore, and Hillary Goulter. I wanted to make sure I wasn't crazy to think this book was almost ready for Kristen, but I also wanted honest feedback if any improvements were needed. I got both, from each of you. Thank you for your valuable feedback, your support, and for helping me reach my publishing goal!

I'd also like to thank everyone I've learned from over the years, everyone who contributed to me sitting here now sharing what I'm sharing in this book—including but not limited to those mentioned in this book, such as Laura Lavigne, Elke Macartney, and Marcia Baczynski.

And thanks to Christine Kloser again, for another round of Get Your Book Done, which helped me get started with this book! *I love your program.*

I'd also like to thank you—you who are reading this right now. Thanks for your interest and for putting the time and energy into reading this book—and hopefully also into implementing at least some of the recommendations I shared. And thanks in advance for telling others about this book! Together, we can make a difference in many lives through the ripple effect.

And finally, thanks to anyone not mentioned here who supported me, encouraged me, or inspired me along the way of this *Detox Your Life* book journey. As I said in the Acknowledgments of *The Multi-Orgasmic Diet,* it takes a village. And, once again, that is true.

Thank you!

ABOUT THE AUTHOR

Rebecca Clio Gould is a holistic health and resilience coach, qigong and meditation teacher, and award-winning author of *The Multi-Orgasmic Diet*. After leaving law school to pursue her passions, she graduated from the Heartwood Institute and then also from the Institute for Integrative Nutrition as a health coach. She is also a certified Sheng Zhen teacher, Supreme Science Qigong teacher, Essence Facilitator, and Sexual Awakening for Women Facilitator. Rebecca has been a board certified holistic health practitioner since 2007, with extensive training in various modalities such as massage, Reiki, shiatsu, breathwork, SomatoEmotional Release Therapy, and traditional Chinese medicine's 5-Element Theory. She's also a certified Mental Health First Aid provider.

Rebecca lives in Seattle, Washington. And when she is not writing, teaching, or working with clients, Rebecca is most likely to be found out in nature or on a comfy couch—enjoying some downtime, relaxing at home or trying her best not to kill her plants (aka, learning how to garden). She also enjoys painting, singing in her car, and spending quality time with her family and friends and her sweet husky shepherd mix, Buddy.

To contact Rebecca, please visit www.rebeccacliogould.com.

WORK WITH REBECCA

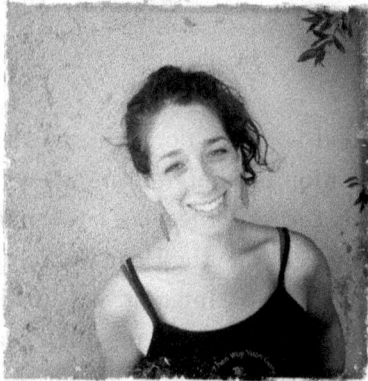

Rebecca's offerings include:

- Meditation and Qigong Classes
- Personalized Guided Meditations
- Holistic Health & Resilience Coaching
- Essence vs Form Sessions
- Magic of Essence Workshops

For more information, freebies, and up-to-date offerings:
www.rebeccacliogould.com

IG: @rebecca.clio.gould and @detox_your_life
FB: @rebeccacliogould and @detoxyourlife

ALSO BY THIS AUTHOR

The Multi-Orgasmic Diet: Embrace Your Sexual Energy and Awaken Your Senses for a Healthier, Happier, Sexier You
by Rebecca Clio Gould

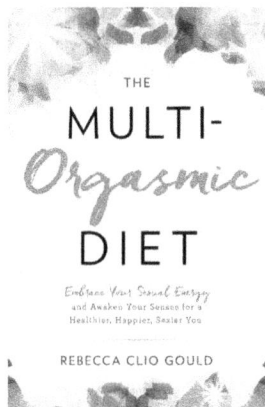

THE

MULTI-
Orgasmic
DIET

Embrace Your Sexual Energy
and Awaken Your Senses for a
Healthier, Happier, Sexier You

REBECCA CLIO GOULD

IPPY AWARD GOLD MEDAL WINNER
Cultivate the power of sexual energy and sensuality to look and feel your best – with over 80 step-by-step practices you can start using today. Plus bonus material!

Don't be fooled by the title. This book doesn't focus on teaching orgasm techniques, and it's not a traditional diet book. It's something better. A sexy spin on diet, weight loss, and women's self-help, *The Multi-Orgasmic Diet* is a revolutionary and fun approach to natural, shame-free healthy living. Instead of a restrictive diet that tells women what to eat and what not to eat, this book provides a lifestyle plan that teaches you how to fill up on the pleasure of life rather than overeating or using emotional eating to fill a void. You will also learn to cultivate deeper love and acceptance for yourself in this body positive approach to women's health and sexuality.

The Multi-Orgasmic Diet gives you:

- A lighthearted, playful, and decidedly sexy way to achieve your weight loss and health goals without restrictions or deprivations.
- A menu plan full of practices to help you cultivate your sexual energy and awaken your senses, both of which will bring more joy and satisfaction to your life.
- A solid foundation that sets you up for success, plus valuable book bonuses and an online community to support you along the way.
- The knowledge you need to use energy cultivation, sensuality, and self-love–not food–for happiness and fulfillment.
- Support in releasing shame and other blockages standing in your way, so that you can live the life of radiant health and happiness you deserve—with sex appeal to boot!
- A pleasure-filled journey that will give you a sexy, alluring glow and spice up your life both in and out of the bedroom.

Learn more at www.rebeccacliogould.com/themod.
Available on Amazon and other major retailers:
amzn.to/2evVgym

ADVANCED PRAISE FOR DETOX YOUR LIFE

"At first I wasn't so sure about this *Detox Your Life* thing, especially the decluttering part. But thanks to this book, I'm no longer sitting in a corner, covered in dust, feeling neglected. My owner took the advice in the Home chapter and gave me away. So now I'm in a new home where I'm loved and played on a regular basis. Thanks, Rebecca Gould. If it weren't for you, I wouldn't have this new and better life! I highly recommend this book."

—1994 Fender Acoustic Guitar

"This book is awesome! Even without going into great detail, you provide great suggestions for how to detox not only your body, but also your mind, your home, and your relationships! I'm honored to be a part of this book. Thank you so much for telling people about me!"

—Chlorella

"The Relationships chapter is my favorite part, but it's all great. I don't really need any of the advice here, but it was cool to see just how well I'm doing without it. I also love how you've helped me understand why some of my exes don't want to talk to me anymore—they're probably narcissists or have borderline personality disorders. So sad."

—The Narcissist

"Until this book came along, I felt so stuck. And I know so many others who have felt this way too. Now I feel so abundant and free! No more stagnation. Everything is flowing great, thanks to this book. A must read! But don't just read it; implement the suggestions. You'll be happy you did.

—Poop

"*Detox Your Life* is a game changer. I used to be a pair of socks, but now I'm a rag. And to be quite honest, I enjoy this role much more. Thanks to Rebecca's advice to get rid of, or repurpose, clothes that have holes in them my life has new meaning now."

—Hole-y Socks-Rag

"Remember that En Vogue song with the lyrics, 'Free your mind, and the rest will follow'? Reading the Mind chapter, I kept hearing "Clean your mind, and the rest will follow"— and it's true. Great advice in that chapter—and all throughout *Detox Your Life*. You will love this book."

—Your Subconscious Mind

www.ingramcontent.com/pod-product-compliance
Lightning Source LLC
Chambersburg PA
CBHW070810280326
41934CB00012B/3139